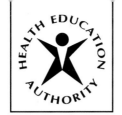

Effectiveness of health promotion interventions in the workplace: a review

Greet Peersman, Angela Harden and Sandy Oliver

**Centre for the Evaluation of Health
Promotion and Social Interventions
Social Science Research Unit
London University Institute of Education**

Series Editor Jane Meyrick

HEA Project Team
Jane Meyrick   Research Project Manager
Antony Morgan   Head of Monitoring and Effectiveness Research

In the same series:
Health promotion in older people for the prevention of coronary heart disease and stroke
Health promotion in childhood and young adolescence for the prevention of unintentional injuries
Effectiveness of video for health education
Effectiveness of mental health promotion interventions
Health promotion with young people for the prevention of substance misuse
Health promotion interventions to promote healthy eating in the general population
Effectiveness of oral health promotion
Effectiveness of interventions to promote healthy eating in preschool children aged 1–5 years: a review
Effectiveness of interventions to promote healthy eating in elderly people living in the community: a review
Effectiveness of interventions to promote healthier living in people from minority ethnic groups: a review
Effectiveness of interventions to promote healthy eating in pregnant women and women of childbearing age: a review
Opportunities for and barriers to change in dietary behaviour in elderly people
Opportunities for and barriers to change in dietary behaviour in minority ethnic groups
Opportunities for and barriers to good nutritional health in women of childbearing age, pregnant women, infants under 1 and children aged 1 to 5

Health Education Authority
Trevelyan House
30 Great Peter Street
London SW1P 2HW

Designed by Edwin Belchamber
Typeset by Wayzgoose
Cover design by Maria Grasso
Printed in Great Britain

Effectiveness of health promotion interventions in the workplace: a review

Contents

Acknowledgements

We would like to acknowledge the invaluable help of Amanda Nicholas, James Thomas, Melanie Mauthner and Ann Oakley at the EPI-Centre.

This report is in part based on a previous systematic review issued by the Social Science Research Unit (SSRU) in 1994 and prepared by the following research team: Merry France-Dawson, Janet Holland, Deirdre Fullerton, Peter Kelley, Sean Arnold and Ann Oakley.

The Centre for the *E*valuation of Health *P*romotion and Social *I*nterventions (EPI-Centre) at the Social Science Research Unit, University of London Institute of Education, is funded by the Department of Health. This grant supports a research team and the development of a specialised computer database (EPIC) compiling bibliographic and methodological details of relevant studies for systematic reviews.

This review was commissioned by the Health Education Authority.

Structure of the report

The report starts with a summary of the main findings from a range of well-designed studies which were identified through extensive literature searches. This is followed by recommendations for future practice and evaluation in the area of workplace health promotion.

The introductory section (Chapter 1) sets out the aims and scope of the review and summarises the methodology used. Chapter 2 describes the policy and research background of workplace health promotion. Chapter 3 provides details on the development, content and delivery of interventions that have been tested by well-designed evaluations for their impact on a range of outcomes, and Chapter 4 reports outcome evaluation studies carried out in the UK.

The discussion in Chapter 5 looks at the rationale for providing health promotion in the workplace-setting in the light of the evidence to date and points to some areas for improvement and future research.

Appendix A describes a framework for the general evaluation of 'social' interventions. Appendix B provides an overview of the review methodology and Appendices C, D, E and F provide further details and the results of each of the different stages of work involved in conducting this review: the identification and classification of relevant studies; the inclusion/exclusion criteria; the assessment of the methodological quality of the studies; and the description of the overall impact of the interventions tested.

Summary tables on the well-designed studies are given in Appendix G in terms of the country where the study was carried out, the population involved, the service provider, the type of workplace, and the objectives and content of the programme, and in Appendix H in terms of the evaluation design.

Finally, included and excluded studies are listed in Appendices I and J, respectively.

Preface

The Health Education Authority (HEA) welcomes this new review of effectiveness of health promotion interventions in the workplace as one means of gathering evidence for health promotion. It forms one of an HEA series of systematic reviews that have begun to address the need for an evidence base in health promotion. This report provides an exhaustive review of the available evidence and highlights the importance for health promoters not only to evaluate their work but to evaluate it well, in order to increase the body of work reviews can draw on. It also highlights the need to consider systematic review evidence alongside other forms of evidence in health promotion work.

The aim of systematic reviews

The commitment within the NHS to move towards evidence-based practice has, to some extent, been mirrored within health promotion. For this reason the methodological tool used to find evidence, the systematic review, has been applied to a range of health promotion topics in an effort to inform health professionals in addition to increasing the knowledge base about effective health promotion.

Executive summary

The workplace has enormous potential as a setting for improving the health of the adult population because of the following: the ease of access to a large number of people, many of whom are at risk for adverse health effects; a potentially high level of participation as programmes are provided on-site; a potentially low level of attrition as the population is relatively stable; cohesion of the working community which can offer benefits such as positive peer pressure and peer support; and established channels of communication, which can be used to publicise programmes, encourage participation and provide feedback.

Workplace health promotion is well established in the USA and the majority of evaluation studies identified for this review were USA-based. Although many workplace health promotion programmes are in progress in the UK, most have either not been formally evaluated or their results have not been published.

The inclusion criteria for this review were developed with the aim of including specifically studies based on participatory methods, as these are considered more likely to be relevant and acceptable; or those that have gathered both process and outcome measures, as these present us with a better picture of whether, and how, the intervention has worked.

We identified a wide variety of programmes which were mainly targeted at the individual level, though some of them were supported by environmental modifications of a varying degree. Overall, the relatively low participation rates were a matter of concern. Most evaluations were considered to be methodologically flawed due to the absence of a control or comparison group. This means that data supporting worksite programmes are still not definitive. In addition, the effectiveness of different approaches to workplace health promotion is likely to be influenced by different organisational cultures and there is insufficient discussion of this in the literature. However, we identified a number of studies from which general pointers to potential success can be derived.

Health promotion programmes to effect change in individual behaviour

Some general principles

- There should be visible and enthusiastic support for, and involvement in, the intervention from top management.

- There should be involvement of employees at all organisational levels in the planning, implementation and activities of the intervention.

- A focus on a definable and modifiable risk factor, which constitutes a priority for the specific worker group, can make an intervention more acceptable to that group of workers and increase their participation.

- Interventions should be tailor-made to the characteristics and needs of the recipients.

- Optimal use of local resources (human, physical, organisational) should be made in organising and implementing the intervention.

- Evaluation should be included as an integral part of any new intervention programme and include a range of outcome and process measures.

Trends in effectiveness

- No clear trends in effectiveness could be identified in relation to certain types of interventions, interventions focusing on particular areas of health, or interventions provided by particular categories of people, therefore conclusions about effectiveness can only be drawn from specific individual studies.

- Comprehensive programmes combining screening and risk assessment with a choice of education programmes and/or environmental changes have been effective; however, with few sound studies to draw on, replicating these interventions cannot guarantee success.

- Least effective have been weight control programmes combining education and financial incentives; sustained weight loss appears particularly difficult and more effort is required to develop and evaluate interventions aimed at long-term weight control.

- There is no conclusive evidence for the effectiveness of social support provided by peers or group leaders as part of broad educational interventions.

- The effect of interventions incorporating a skill development component is inconclusive with equal numbers of effective and ineffective interventions; however, combining skills training with social support in interventions targeting a specific risk behaviour is more likely to be effective than skills training as part of broad complex interventions.

- Healthier eating has been encouraged by targeted provision of information, such as point-of-purchase labelling of healthy food choices in the workplace cafetaria, and computer-generated personalised nutrition advice.

- Two complex interventions addressing healthy eating were considered ineffective: one operated at the level of individuals, organisations and communities; the other involved presentations, computerised data analysis, supermarket tours, take-home activities and group walks.

- Individualised delivery of information appeared effective in a range of interventions. This finding was also supported by a process evaluation of a complex intervention suggesting that engaging the 'eager' employees into wellness programmes was easy if programmes were provided on-site; engaging the 'reluctant' employees required one-to-one approaches.

- The importance of healthy alliances was supported by a number of studies showing success in controlling blood pressure, smoking and alcohol consumption, as well as improving knowledge and changing behaviour related to cancer prevention; however, other studies involving healthy alliances had disappointing results.

Recommendations for developing and implementing interventions

- Interventions should be targeted at specific groups at risk of particular health hazards and tailor-made with the characteristics and needs of those groups in mind.

- In addition to opportunist use of the workplace for health promotion interventions addressing broader public health needs, attention must be paid to the short-term and long-term health dangers imposed by conditions in the workplace.

- Workplace health promotion strategies should not isolate health-related knowledge, values and behaviours from the social and material context in which the targeted employees live.

- Organisations should employ both population-based policy initiatives and intensive individually- and group-oriented health promotion interventions to create an integrated programme for change.

- A sustained programme based on principles of empowerment and/or a community-oriented model using multiple methods, visibly supported by top management and engaging the involvement of all levels of workers in an organisation, is likely to produce the best results.

Recommendations for evaluating interventions

- Interventions with multiple components should be clearly described in terms of what these components are, how they are implemented and by whom.

- Workplace health promotion interventions should have fully integrated evaluation components initially focusing on the delivery and acceptability of the interventions and ultimately addressing their effectiveness.

- Appropriate quantitative and qualitative procedures, as well as statistical techniques for analysing effectiveness, should be used.

- Where feasible, studies of effectiveness should employ the design of a randomised controlled trial, although quasi-experimental approaches with adequate control or comparison groups should also be considered.

- Evaluations of workplace health promotion interventions should include systematic information on cost-effectiveness where possible.

- The need for methodological rigour must be recognised among evaluators of health promotion activities, and among peer reviewers and editors of journals to raise publication standards, including the importance of publishing studies reporting 'negative' results.

- The widespread lack of methodological rigour requires commissioners and providers to use information from systematic reviews or from critically appraised primary studies to plan their services.

- There is a need to develop research methods appropriate for evaluating the role of healthy alliances and other complex interventions with the aim to assess their effectiveness and to identify their active components.

1. Introduction

Aims

The aims of the review described in this report were:
- To locate and describe available evaluations of interventions aimed at promoting the health of the employed population.

- To undertake a critical review of the quality of these interventions, focusing on the ways in which they have been evaluated and the conclusions about their effect that can reliably be drawn from them.

- To summarise the state-of-the-art with respect to implementing and evaluating different approaches to promoting people's health at work, and to indicate future research, policy and practice needs.

The review considers two basic questions:
1. How do we know what works in the field of social and behavioural interventions?
2. What evidence is there for the effectiveness of different interventions?

Scope of the review

Reports informing the development and evaluation of interventions targeted at people in the workplace setting were sought. The focus was on interventions promoting risk reduction *behaviours* relevant to the prevention of disease and the promotion of healthy lifestyles. Evaluation reports of interventions were included only if they aimed either directly (at the individual level) or indirectly (at the organisational level) at behaviour change. Thus interventions which involved organisational modification with no implications for behaviour change were excluded. Evaluations of interventions *exclusively* focusing on smoking were excluded to avoid duplication of effort with the Review Group on Tobacco Control of the Cochrane Collaboration, an international effort to promote evidence-based health care. This group prepares and maintains systematic reviews on smoking prevention and cessation disseminated through the Cochrane Library, which is available on CD-ROM as well as on-line (Cochrane Library 1998).

For health promotion interventions to be both necessary and relevant, they should be based on a needs assessment and developed by involving the people for whom they are intended. At the very least, programmes should be piloted and their content and delivery amended according to the participants' views before an extensive outcome evaluation is undertaken. To maximise learning from evaluations, they should ideally include a range of process and outcome measures.

We restricted the inclusion of studies to outcome evaluations of interventions that were based on a needs assessment and/or developed using participatory methods and/or previously piloted with the study/target population, and/or outcome evaluations that included at least one process measure other than programme reach or monitoring of intervention implementation.

To maximise the validity of the review conclusions, retrospective studies were excluded. In addition, the methodological quality of prospective evaluation studies was assessed for the presence/absence of four minimum quality criteria with the aim to identify the subset of studies from which potentially reliable conclusions can be drawn. These 'sound' studies are discussed in detail in Chapter 3. Since the impact of interventions assessed by 'flawed' evaluations is unclear, a detailed description of these studies falls outside the scope of this review. We have, however, made an exception for studies carried out in the UK. These are described in Chapter 4, but caution has to be taken in drawing conclusions from these studies as none met the minimum quality criteria for a 'sound' evaluation.

Methodology

A full description of the methodology used in this review is provided in Appendices B and C.

The main aim of the literature searches was to identify outcome evaluations of health promotion interventions in the workplace published since an earlier review by Frances-Dawson et al. (1994). The bibliography of the studies covered in the previous report was extended by systematic hand searches, electronic database searches, scanning the reference lists of reports of relevant outcome evaluation studies and through personal contacts (see 'Search strategies' in Appendix C).

The search results were subsequently entered/downloaded into BiblioMap, the EPI-Centre bibliographic register of health promotion studies. We used the EPI-Centre standardised coding strategy to classify all reports according to the type of study, the country where the study was carried out, the health focus, the study population and, in case of intervention studies, also for the type of intervention and the intervention provider (see 'Search results' in Appendix C).

All outcome evaluations for which the full report could be obtained within the time limit set for the review, were screened according to the inclusion/exclusion criteria and included studies further assessed for the presence/absence of four minimum methodological qualities (see Appendices B and E). Two reviewers independently assessed each study and any disagreements were discussed and resolved with a third reviewer, if necessary. A final element in the reviewing process consisted of judging the effectiveness of the programme from the information provided in the published reports, and bearing in mind the 'quality' attributes referred to above. These reviewers' assessments of effectiveness were then contrasted with those provided by the authors themselves (see Appendices E and F). The resulting subset of studies from which potentially reliable conclusions can be drawn, were described and discussed in terms of effectiveness (see Chapter 3). Recommendations were made for developing and implementing interventions and for evaluating interventions in the workplace setting.

The approaches used in this review follow the model for reviewing health care interventions established in the Cochrane Collaboration (Cochrane Collaboration, 1994), and the work of other reviewers in the health, education and social welfare fields (Biglan *et al.*, 1987; Chalmers and Haynes, 1994; Dickersin and Lefebvre, 1994; Knipschild, 1994; Loevinsohn, 1990; MacDonald, Sheldon and Gillespie, 1992; Mulrow, 1994; Schnaps *et al.*, 1981; Schwartz, Flamant and Lellouch, 1980). The methods used in the present report have been applied in a range of systematic reviews conducted by the SSRU and the EPI-Centre looking at the ways in which health promotion and other social interventions have been evaluated and what we can learn from them (France-Dawson *et al.*, 1994; Fullerton and Oakley, 1995; Oakley and Fullerton, 1994; Oakley, Fullerton and Holland, 1995; Oakley *et al.*, 1994a,b, 1995a,b, 1996; Peersman *et al.*, 1996).

2. Background

Over the last decade health promotion, with its focus on the facilitation of healthy lifestyles by altering both people's environments and their individual behaviour, has become a central feature of health policy at local, national and international levels. Health promotion is often thought of as a 'new' concept. However, some argue that it is merely a 'renaissance' of a broad and encompassing concept of public health (Green and Kreuter, 1991). Efforts to control rising health care costs·by decreasing the need for medical care provided an initial boost for a renewed interest in health promotion. The epidemiological revolution of chronic diseases and the realisation that many of their risk factors are preventable and not amenable to improvement by medicine, the ageing of the population, the widening social class gradient in health, and pressure from health lobby groups further supported the development of a health promotion policy (Clark and McLeroy, 1995; Green and Kreuter, 1991; Hawe, Degeling and Hall, 1995; Pencak, 1991; Wong, Alsagoff and Koh, 1992). Coronary heart disease (CHD), stroke and cancers account for 65% of all deaths in England (OPCS, 1992; Townsend and Davidson, 1986; Townsend, Davidson and Whitehead, 1988; Whitehead, 1987). In 1988, 19 948 men and 5535 women between the ages of 15 and 64 died from CHD in England. Lung and breast cancer are important causes of premature death in women (ASH, 1993; OPCS, 1992). Considerable variation in mortality, in the prevalence of risk factors and in the uptake of preventive health care services between different geographic regions, and within different neighbourhoods or ethnic groups have been described (Townsend and Davidson, 1986; Whitehead, 1987). Risk factors include smoking; elevated cholesterol levels and blood pressure; an unhealthy diet; diabetes; obesity; lack of physical exercise; and certain psycho-social factors.

Why health promotion in the workplace?

Almost half the UK population is employed and individuals may spend up to 60% of their waking hours in their place of work. Workplace accidents and illness are a considerable burden; their overall cost to the British economy is estimated to be between £6 billion and £13 billion (i.e. 1–2% of gross domestic product) (Faculty of Public Health Medicine, 1995). The workplace is therefore considered an important determinant of health and influence on lifestyle. There are several reasons why it is a popular setting for health promotion initiatives: it provides easy and regular access to a large number of people who make up a relatively stable population, so repeated interventions are feasible; it has the potential for higher participation rates than in 'non-captive' situations, and employers can often be persuaded to offer incentives to increase participation; it may encourage sustained peer support and positive peer pressure; and it provides access to young men, who have particularly low general practitioner (GP) consultation rates, and are thus unlikely to benefit from opportunistic health promotion activity in primary care designed to increase awareness of health issues and help to establish healthier behaviours (Faculty of Public Health Medicine, 1995).

Workplace health promotion has been associated with a reduction in health risks and promotion of healthy lifestyles; and with improvements in economic and productivity factors including medical costs, compensation benefits, employee absenteeism, job satisfaction and productivity (Alexy, 1991; Goetzel *et al.*, 1996; Knight *et al.*, 1994; Sapolsky *et al.*, 1981). Workplace health promotion also has the potential to be actively disseminated by employees to their families and social networks, thus having an indirect effect on the health of the community at large (Faculty of Public Health Medicine, 1995).

Participation in workplace health promotion

To serve disease prevention purposes effectively, worksite health promotion programmes need to attract a large proportion of eligible employees. Larger worksites tend to carry out more health promotion activities than smaller sites (Fielding and Piserchia, 1989), but smaller sites have been shown to be more likely to have higher rates of employee participation (Glasgow *et al.*, 1990). Reported estimates of participation rates in workplace health promotion programmes ranged from 20 to 60% (Heaney and Inglish, 1995).

Although overall participation rates are important, to gain the most benefit in terms of disease prevention, employees who are at risk of adverse health outcomes particularly need to participate. However, studies suggest that smokers, hypertensives, employees with elevated cholesterol levels, and those who lead sedentary lifestyles are less likely to join (Heany and Inglish, 1995). Participants are more likely to be younger; well-educated, female (except for exercise programmes); non-smokers; and white-collar workers (Alexy, 1991; Gebhardt and Crump, 1990; Greene and Strychar, 1992; Sorensen, Pechacek and Pallonen, 1986; Spilman, 1988; Stunkard, Cohen and Felix, 1989; Zavela *et al.*, 1988). Workplace health promotion initiatives are less likely to reach low earners and those who are intermittently employed (Faculty of Public Health Medicine, 1995).

Studies also suggest that participation rates differ according to the focus of the programme. Spilman (1988) found that women participated in weight reduction programmes regardless of whether or not they were overweight. Davis *et al.* (1987) found that people who were at higher risk for particular factors were more likely to participate in certain health promotion activities, such as weight loss and stress control, but not others such as alcohol prevention or exercise programmes.

In an evaluation of a community project to reduce nutrition-related risk of cancer, Potter *et al.* (1990) used a 'benefits and barriers scale' to describe different groups of participants. There were four groups, those who: (1) saw diet as having a large effect on health and perceived dietary change as easy (i.e. high benefits; low barriers); (2) felt that while diet affected health, the required dietary changes were difficult (high benefits; high barriers); (3) perceived diet as having little effect, but that change would not be difficult (low benefits; low barriers); and (4) did not think diet mattered and would find changes too difficult (low benefits; high barriers).

Participation rates have been said to be increased by the use of incentives, social support and management support (Baranowski *et al.*, 1990; Erfurt *et al.*, 1990; Glasgow, McCaul and Fisher, 1993; Stachnik and Stoffelmayr, 1983). Glasgow *et al.* (1993) suggested that in addition to involving top management and union representatives in publicising health programmes, the use of repeated promotions and multiple communication channels could enhance participation. They also suggested combining these with the involvement of enthusiastic employees, the identification of subgroups unlikely to participate and the devotion of adequate time, money and effort to promote the programme.

Types of programmes

Workplace health promotion interventions tend to fit into one of three categories (O'Donnell, 1987; Pencak, 1991):

(1) *Awareness* programmes aim to increase the participants' level of awareness in relation to a particular health area. Activities include: health fairs; posters; newsletters; educational classes; and health screening. Participants are expected to make changes in health behaviour as a result of increased awareness.

(2) *Lifestyle change* programmes are aimed directly at changing employees' health behaviour using a variety of strategies such as

skills training and self-help.

(3) *Supportive environment* programmes aim to promote a sustainable, healthy lifestyle through creating a workplace environment that supports and encourages healthy choices, such as a smoking ban and the provision of healthy food choices in the canteen. Examples of programmes including these environmental modifications are: Look After Your Heart and the Welsh Heart Programme (Heartbeat Wales) in the UK; Live for Life, Minnesota Heart Program and Total Life Concept in the USA (Reason, 1989; Nutbeam and Catford, 1987; Wilbur, 1983; Mittelmark *et al.*, 1989, respectively).

The British experience

In 1974, the Health and Safety at Work Act suggested that working environments should be safe, not placing the workforce in any situation which is detrimental to good health. As implementation of the Act was not widespread, further government recommendations were considered in 1984, and outlined in a code of practice (Clarkson and Blower, 1991; Jacobsen, Smith and Whitehead, 1991).

In 1989, the Labour Research Department reported the findings from a survey of 500 trade union representatives. The most common workplace health promotion activities cited were first aid/medical treatment, inspection of hazards and pre-employment medical screening (Labour Research Department, 1989). Activities union representatives wished to target included stress management, breast screening and screening for hypertension.

A survey of 1344 workplaces conducted in 1992 by the Health Education Authority (HEA) found that 40% undertook at least one major health-related activity in the previous year. The likelihood of this increased with workplace size. The workplaces of foreign-owned companies were more likely to have health promotional activity than British-owned ones. The presence of a recognised union was another important factor – for example, 41% of workplaces with a recognised union had a smoking-related activity, compared to 28% without a union. Workplaces with no health promotion activity were virtually all small- or medium-sized, in the private sector, British-owned, and predominantly in the distribution and catering business. The main reasons given for not undertaking such activities were: being too small (55%); too busy (11%); not necessary (9%); or not worth doing (9%). Health issues were rated very highly as a workplace issue (41–69%), with smoking being considered most important (25–52%); although over 80% of employees were in relatively sedentary jobs, exercise was not rated very highly. The range of health-related activities was very large; while action on smoking was the most common, there was also considerable activity in the areas of alcohol abuse, stress, and HIV/AIDS; and in larger workplaces on heart health, weight control, exercise and fitness. Although workplaces that have a preponderance of female employees were more likely to have breast and cervical cancer screening facilities, there was little difference in the overall general levels of activity compared with predominantly male workplaces. The main implementation method was through group communication such as posters, leaflets, video; larger workplaces were considerably more likely to offer counselling for smoking cessation, alcohol abuse and stress. There was no evidence that budgets for health promotion activity were routinely available, though larger workplaces were more likely to have either a personnel executive or occupational health nurse/doctor, whereas in other workplaces responsibility was taken by someone with no specific training or qualification in this area. There was very little formal evaluation of the programmes; assessment largely happened through informal feedback from the workforce. Whilst there was support for the aims of health promotion and positive advantages were perceived, there was little evidence of institutionalisation of the activities into the culture of the workplace (HEA, 1993).

Overall, the UK lags behind other countries in both the extent and provision of programmes and in evaluating such programmes (Sanders and Crowe, 1996). It has been suggested that this is due to the fact that occupational health services are not a statutory part of the National Health Service, unlike in other countries (Labour Research Department, 1989; Fielding, 1990; Jacobsen, Smith and Whitehead, 1991).

The *health of the nation* white paper produced by the government in 1992 described the workplace as an important arena for developing health promotion interventions. It stated:

> The increasing concern of employers and their workforces to improve health opens major opportunities to develop and increase activity on general health promotion in the workplace. The Government will set up a task force to examine and develop activity on health promotion in the workplace. The Departments of Health and Employment, the Health and Safety Executive, the Health Education Authority, representatives from Wider Health Working, the Confederation of British Industry, the Trades Union Congress and other business organisations will be invited to join. The objective will be to advise on new initiatives, including health promotion campaigns and on materials which can be produced for the workplace. (Department of Health, 1992, p. 28)

The National Health Service (NHS) received some encouragement for implementing workplace health promotion:

> The NHS must set an example to other employers and show what can be achieved. The NHS Management Executive has set up a task group of NHS managers, HEA representatives and professionals to review the way in which the NHS promotes the health of its own employees. The group will bring forward proposals for national and local targets, including proposals for units, health centres, GP practices and other workplaces in the NHS to declare themselves 'healthy workplaces'. (Department of Health, 1992, p. 36)

The *health of the nation* targets a number of key areas in which 'effective interventions should be possible' including CHD and stroke, cancer and accidents. With these targets in mind, the HEA prioritised the development and support for health promotion in the workplace over a five-year period to include: Look After Your Heart, Cancer Education, Smoking Education, Alcohol Education and Nutrition Education (Hagard, Chambers and Killoran, 1991).

The American experience

Several factors influenced the creation of workplace health promotion programmes in the USA. These included the rising costs of health care for corporations, which contribute around 30% of the national health care bill by providing medical insurance to around 80% of their workforces and their families as an employee benefit (Conrad, 1988; Wong, Alsagoff and Koh, 1992). By 1984, American employers paid over $90 billion in employee health insurance. In addition to the obvious economic benefits, health promotion programmes offer other potential benefits to employers and their staff. They may improve the employer's image, as concern for employees' health and wellbeing are highly valued by society (Pencak, 1991). They may also enhance the recruitment of 'fitter' staff through their interest in health issues, and increase employee morale and job commitment (Baun, Bernacki and Tsai, 1986; Sapolsky *et al.*, 1981; Weinstein, 1983), which in turn may result in less absenteeism due to ill health and improved productivity (Cox, Shephard and Corey, 1981; Foshee *et al.*, 1986).

In 1980, the first Surgeon General's report on health promotion and disease prevention entitled *Objectives for the nation* targeted fifteen objectives for health promotion activities including smoking cessation, reducing misuse of alcohol and drugs, improved nutrition, exercise and fitness and stress control (Castillo-Salgado, 1984; DHHS, 1980).

The American public health movement has, however, been deeply divided with regard to where the emphasis should be placed in the effort to promote workers' health (Walsh *et al.*, 1991). Occupational health specialists locate the core problem in the design of plants and jobs, while the behavioural sciences emphasise personal risk factors that may be exacerbated by job conditions or may be particularly amenable to interventions at work, but are fundamentally an individual affair. Walsh *et al.* (1991) found that workers did not believe that health risks associated with their lifestyle or job can simply be seen as a matter of individual control, nor can they be stripped entirely of personal responsibility.

Hollander and Lengermann (1988) assessed the nature and extent of health promotion programmes in Fortune 500 companies, seen to be a good barometer of the 'state-of-the-art' in the work setting because of their large number of employees, their interest in cost savings, and their track record of investing in innovative programmes. They found that higher ranked, larger and high technology companies were more likely to have health promotion programmes; to offer more diverse activities; to have plans for programme expansion; to use models of cost-sharing and company time to participate; to make greater use of health professionals; and to use needs assessment, evaluation and cost-analysis techniques.

Worksite health promotion often follows a set pattern beginning with an assessment of the employees' health risks. For example, the Total Life Concept programme conducts a health risk appraisal followed by various lifestyle improvement modules on exercise, back pain, weight control, high blood pressure, stress management, smoking cessation, nutrition, etc. (Ingledew, 1986). Health Risk Appraisal (HRA) is a common component of workplace health promotion and essentially consists of: (1) an assessment of personal health habits and risk factors; (2) an estimation of the individual's future risk of death and/or adverse health outcomes from several specific causes; and (3) the provision of educational messages and/or counselling about ways to change one or several personal risk factors that might lower personal risk of death or disease (Boudreau *et al.*, 1995). HRA has become increasingly sophisticated and often includes measures of mental and social, as well as physical wellbeing. Data from the National Survey of Workplace Health Promotion Activities in the USA showed that, in 1989, 29.5% of the worksites in the private sector had provided HRA activities with larger worksites being more often involved in these activities. Despite considerable investment in the development, dissemination and use of HRA, there is only limited empirical evidence that these have any effect on behaviour modification and results are generally inconclusive. The most positive reports of the effects on behaviour change come from studies which do not use no-intervention control groups (Boudreau *et al.*, 1995).

3. The methodologically sound studies

We assessed a total of 139 separate outcome evaluation studies for inclusion in this review. Of these, 89 (64%) did not match our inclusion criteria. A comparison between the scope of included and excluded studies showed that, overall, the inclusion/exclusion criteria employed did not result in bias towards inclusion of studies in a particular health area or of a particular intervention type only (see Appendix D).

Fifty (36%) studies matched the inclusion criteria, and were further assessed for their methodological quality with the aim of identifying the subset from which potentially reliable conclusions can be drawn. Only 15 (30%) of these were judged to be methodologically 'sound' (see Appendix E). The sound studies are starred twice (**) when referred to in the text, the flawed studies are starred once (*).

Twelve sound studies were carried out in the USA, one in Canada, one involved worksites in both the USA and Canada, and one study was carried out in the Netherlands. Three of the interventions tested in those studies were broad health promotion programmes including cardiovascular screening and risk assessment (**Erfurt et al., 1991a (3024); **Kronenfeld et al., 1987 (3019); **Wilbur, Hartwell and Piserchia, 1986 (3074)); two focused on weight loss (**Forster, Jeffery and Snell, 1988 (3066); **Jeffery, Forster and Snell, 1985 (3067)); one combined weight loss with smoking (**Jeffery et al., 1993 (3006)); four focused on healthy eating (**Levin, 1996 (3088); **Brug et al., 1996 (3093); **Sorensen et al., 1996 (3135); **Sheeshka and Woolcott, 1994 (3148)); one combined healthy eating with smoking (**Glasgow et al., 1994 (3007)); two interventions targeted alcohol abuse (**Stoltzfus and Benson, 1994 (3126); **Cook, Back and Trudeau, 1996 (3143)); one focused on osteoporosis (**Brown, 1996 (3089)); and one aimed at reducing occupational cancer (**Parkinson et al., 1989 (3030)).
Note: Numbers following the studies refer to the unique identification number of the report on EPIC, the effectiveness database of the EPI-Centre.

Descriptions of the sound studies are given below under the headings related to the main focus of the intervention: cardiovascular screening and risk assessment; weight loss; healthy eating; alcohol abuse; and osteoporosis. Several of the studies involved participants in developing and/or delivering the intervention and they are discussed further under 'Healthy alliances'. Summaries of the interventions and the evaluation designs of these studies are given in Appendices G and H, respectively.

The assessments of the effects of interventions noted are those of the reviewers. Interventions are judged as effective, effective for some groups only, ineffective or harmful in terms of the outcomes intended to be measured. The main reason for judging the effect of an intervention as unclear was a high attrition rate (i.e. a third or more) not adequately dealt with (for example, no information on those who dropped out was provided).

Cardiovascular screening and risk assessment

Screening and/or risk assessment exercises introduced employees to three different comprehensive interventions focusing on cardiovascular health (**Erfurt *et al.*, 1991a (3024); **Kronenfeld *et al.*, 1987 (3019); **Wilbur, Hartwell and Piserchia, 1986 (3074).

In a study comparing health promotion interventions varying in intensity, four worksites were randomly assigned to one of four conditions (**Erfurt *et al.*, 1991 (3024)). Site 1 offered screening with referral to treatment/wellness programmes for those who had cardiovascular disease risks. Site 2, in addition, provided health education and twice-yearly health improvement classes, testing the underlying assumption that people will make health behaviour changes if they have both proper information about their current health status, and ways to learn how to make appropriate behaviour changes. At Site 3, health education interventions identical to those offered at Site 2 were combined with outreach and follow-up counselling. Employees with one or more of the targeted cardiovascular risk factors were contacted about once every six months, counselled about their current risk status, and assisted in exploring how they might change. A menu approach to wellness interventions was offered, including guided self-help, one-to-one formal consultation, interactive small group interventions, or formal group sessions. The underlying assumption tested here, was that behaviour change does not only require information but also needs support, encouragement, and assistance in problem-solving along with a broad range of service types. Programme interventions were most comprehensive at Site 4, which also included social organisations such as the creation of informal health networks and peer support groups; walking clubs; weight loss contests; and plant-wide 'smoke-outs'. This approach emphasised encouraging people to improve their health by adopting positive substitutes for behaviours that create long-term health risks. See also 'Healthy alliances'.

An integral process evaluation found that engaging the 'eager' employees into wellness programmes was easy if programmes were provided on-site; engaging the 'reluctant' employees required one-to-one approaches and the provision of increased choice through a menu approach. At the end of the three-year study period, Sites 3 and 4, which included outreach and counselling, had engaged about 46% of identified smokers in smoking cessation activities and 54% of those who were overweight in weight loss activities. This compared to a participation rate of less than 10% at Site 2, and less than 1% at Site 1. The authors concluded that offering a menu of activities even though they were offered outside working hours, was more successful in increasing participation than offering only health education classes. Offering activities on company time might have increased participation, but would also have increased cost (★★Erfurt *et al.*, 1991a (3024)).

Some health improvements occurred at all four sites, but the more intensive programmes (Sites 3 and 4) were more effective in reducing smoking and controlling blood pressure. Overall, the intervention appeared ineffective for weight loss as the weight lost by some people was offset by the weight gained by others. Maintenance of improvements in risk factors was related to those programmes including continuing follow-up counselling (★★Erfurt *et al.*, 1991a (3024)).

A cost-effectiveness analysis of this study indicated that Sites 3 and 4 were nine to ten times more cost-effective in engaging employees into programme participation; and five to six times more cost-effective in reducing risks/preventing relapse as compared to Site 2. The total direct cost per per cent of risks reduced/relapse prevented was less than one dollar per employee per year. However, the authors indicated that programme costs may vary considerably across companies because of differences in salary structures and overhead costs (★★Erfurt, Foote and Heirich, 1992 (3061)).

Carolina Healthstyle (★★Kronenfeld *et al.*, 1987 (3019)), a state-funded comprehensive health promotion project, focused on South Carolina state employees. The programme was evaluated by comparing the health behaviour and health attitudes of employees at 18 state agencies which formed the first implementation wave, with those of employees in other agencies which started the project at a later stage.

The project started with promotional activities such as films, lunchtime presentations, and a Health Risk Appraisal. The intervention agencies formed healthstyle committees which selected a series of programmes of interest in various aspects of health behaviour change (see also 'Healthy alliances'). Programmes typically included weight control and nutrition, stress management, exercise, smoking cessation, alcohol education and safety education. Some agencies also offered first aid courses, and talks on the use of health care. Along with encouraging changes at the individual level, the project tried to encourage changes at the policy level with respect to smoking, seat-belt use, and the inclusion of nutritious food in snack bars. Posters and bulletin boards were used to encourage various positive health practices, for example food choices in the cafeteria, and using stairs rather than elevators. Certain activities were provided to all state agencies whether part of the intervention group or not. These included a quarterly newsletter, twice-yearly walking events, and a field day providing health information sessions and encouraging physical activity.

Ten months after initial programme implementation, the intervention was deemed effective in reducing the level of alcohol consumption, both in terms of increasing the proportion of very moderate drinkers and reducing the number of binge drinking episodes. There were small but non-significant positive changes in the proportion of employees smoking and a significant decline in the percentage of heavy smokers (i.e. more than 30 cigarettes a day) at the intervention agencies. However, interpretation of these changes was complicated by the fact that there were some significant differences in smoking habits between intervention and comparison agencies at baseline. The reviewers therefore judged the intervention unclear in its effect on smoking. Intervention agencies were not significantly different from comparison agencies in exercise behaviour, in dietary habits (i.e. the consumption of saturated fats, vegetables and desserts), in safety practices (i.e. the use of seat belts and infant restraints), and in stress or other mental health measures.

By the end of 1984, the Live For Life programme (**Wilbur, Hartwell and Piserchia, 1986 (3074)) was available to more than 25 000 Johnson & Johnson employees at 43 locations in the USA, Puerto Rico, Canada and Europe. The long-term aim of the programme was to help contain health care costs attributable to unhealthy lifestyles that are amenable to modification in the work setting. Specific programme objectives were to improve health knowledge, physical fitness, and nutrition; to control weight, stress, blood pressure, and alcohol consumption; to stop smoking; and to use medical services appropriately.

A programme coordinator was assigned to each participating company to ensure that the project was adequately planned, organised and implemented. Volunteers from middle- and upper management level acted as leaders during the programme start-up and worked closely with a cross-section of employees in different task forces addressing key areas of health (see also 'Healthy alliances'). Most of the participants took part in a health screen including clinical risk factors as well as behavioural and attitudinal measures. The results were fed back by means of an attractive document, the Lifestyle Profile, in the context of a three-hour lifestyle seminar. Personal responsibility for health was emphasised and health-enhancing programme opportunities were promoted. Intensive action programmes (i.e. 4–12 sessions) focused on aerobic exercise; weight control through a reduction in calorie intake and regular exercise; healthy eating patterns; smoking cessation; stress management through mental and physical relaxation, and improved personal assertiveness; blood pressure control; reduction in alcohol consumption; and yoga. Shorter programmes were available on breast self-examination, bio-feedback, nutrition, blood pressure, and carbon monoxide analysis for smokers.

A high employee participation rate was achieved through the provision of regular and convenient programmes in combination with environmental changes such as the provision of on-site exercise facilities with showers and lockers; scales in rest-rooms; nutritious foods in the cafeteria and vending machines; self-administered blood pressure equipment; as well as car-pooling; a smoking policy; the organisation of health fairs; and the provision of incentive prizes and awards for participation in Live For Life activities. Participation in the health screen represented 73–79% of the total employee population; those who took part were relatively young, fairly healthy and fairly highly educated.

The programme was evaluated by comparing four intervention sites with three control sites in the USA. Preliminary results comparing baseline with health screen measures one year later showed significant improvements in fitness, smoking, stress management, weight control and employee attitudes (i.e. self-reported sick days, satisfaction with working conditions and with personal relations at work, ability to handle job strain, job self-esteem).

Weight loss

Sound evaluations of weight control programmes suggest that this is a particularly challenging goal for health promotion interventions.

Two similar interventions combining education with financial incentives collected through payroll deduction were evaluated (**Forster *et al.*, 1985 (3066); **Jeffery, Forster and Snell, 1985 (3067)).

The programme tested in the study by **Jeffery, Forster and Snell, 1985 (3067), required university employees to set their own weight reduction goals which could range from weight maintenance to a maximum of 24% of initial body weight over 6 months (i.e. 1% per week). Participation in activities was optional and included 2-weekly weigh-ins and group educational sessions, and homework assignments based on a weight loss manual and records for monitoring eating habits. The approach emphasised gradual changes in diet towards a lower calorie intake, increased energy expenditure through moderate-intensity physical activity such as walking, and systematic modification of social and environmental factors to support behaviour change. Participants agreed to have a fixed amount withheld from their pay cheque. If weight loss was slower than specified in their incentive plan or a scheduled weigh-in was missed, payroll deduction money was retained but could be earned back depending on progress made at later weigh-ins. Money remaining after the last weigh-in was divided among those who achieved their personal weight loss goals.

Only 36 individuals representing 6% of the eligible population, participated. They were randomly assigned to an intervention or control group. After 3 months, weight loss was significantly higher in the intervention group as compared to the control group. The programme was then also implemented in the control group. Comparing the total weight loss for the two groups over 6 months showed that participants in the delayed-intervention group lost more than twice as much weight as those in the early-intervention condition. The authors suggested potential reasons for this observation: a seasonal or holiday effect; having had more time to prepare for participation; more efficient intervention provision; and/or higher levels of mutual interaction and support among participants in the delayed-intervention group. Interest in continuing the programme beyond the initial 6-month period was related to initial success in weight loss. However, follow-up data suggested that most of the weight lost was regained within one year after the intervention finished. The authors concluded that without continued intervention, worksites do not appear to offer special advantages in aiding weight control (**Forster, Jeffery and Snell, 1988 (3055)). The reviewers judged this intervention to be effective in the short-term only.

A variation of the above intervention was evaluated by **Forster *et al.*, 1985 (3066) in a 2 x 2 factorial design. Programmes differed by whether group instructional sessions were offered on an optional or required basis, and whether or not financial incentives were split between attendance at fortnightly weigh-ins and weight loss, or were received for weight loss alone. The instructional sessions aimed to reinforce the messages in the self-instruction manual and were led by a health educator who also offered advice for individual problems. Though both men and women were more likely to agree to participate in programmes not offering classes, required attendance at scheduled events seemed especially unattractive to men. Weight loss was highest among those using self-instruction in combination with financial incentives for weight loss. However, group differences were not statistically significant and the study lacked a no-intervention control group. Pooled follow-up data (**Forster, Jeffery and Snell, 1988 (3055)) suggested that most of the weight lost was regained within a year. Again, the interventions tested were effective in the short-term only.

The disappointing results from the studies discussed above, were confirmed in an evaluation of a similar intervention, the Healthy Worker Project, targeting both weight control and smoking cessation (**Jeffery, Forster and French, 1993 (3006)). Thirty-two worksites were randomised to an intervention or control group. The intervention consisted of health education classes combined with a payroll-based incentive system. Four rounds of 11 weekly sessions each were offered on-site over 2 years and covered behaviour modification principles for weight loss and for smoking cessation. Classes were held during employee time and repeated several times to accommodate for shift workers. Of a total of 10 000 employees in the intervention worksites, 2041 (20%) participated in the weight control programme and 270 (3%) in smoking cessation activities.

Outcome measurements were based on both cohort and cross-sectional surveys. Allowing for recruitment and attrition rates, net reductions in smoking prevalence over 2 years in intervention compared with control sites were 4.0% and 2.1% in cross-sectional and cohort surveys, respectively. No intervention effect was found for weight. The authors concluded that the smoking programme only could be justified on the grounds of cost-effectiveness (**Jeffery, Forster and French, 1993 (3006)). However, not all relevant factors were addressed in this study: the existence of smoking policies in some sites and not others was not accounted for at the time of randomisation, and at some sites smoking policies were introduced during the two years of the intervention (Jeffery et al., 1994), which may have interfered with the intervention impact on smoking. The reviewers therefore judged the intervention to be ineffective for weight control and unclear for smoking behaviour.

Healthy eating

The study by **Levin, 1996 (3088), was a point-of-purchase intervention implemented in an urban worksite cafeteria to promote healthy food choices. Three low-fat meals (bean burritos; potato and chilli burritos; turkey, lettuce and tomato sandwich) were labelled with a heart symbol on the menu board and a poster was placed at the entrance to the cafeteria reading 'Look out for the "symbol of a heart" for your low-fat entree selection'. A prize draw for a cookery book took place every week during the 4-week intervention period. Questionnaires were used as raffle tickets and could be entered by any customer regardless of having bought a targeted meal. The sales of targeted meals was monitored by using computerised cash receipts over a period of 4 weeks and compared to the sales of a carefully matched control cafeteria. The latter had identical meals on the menu but no poster or labels to draw attention to the low-fat meals.

Sales of the low-fat meals increased significantly in the intervention cafeteria as compared to the control cafeteria over the 4-week assessment period. Increased sales were maintained at 6 months follow-up, however, since no sales data were collected in the control cafeteria, it is not possible to draw conclusions on the maintenance of dietary intake changes.

This intervention was low-effort, low-budget and relatively easy to monitor. There were no significant differences in age, gender or ethnicity between customers who believed the labels influenced their food choice, which suggests that the intervention is applicable to a variety of groups. In addition, the author indicated that nutrition interventions generally rely on written material which may be difficult to understand. As no other written materials but a poster with minimal wording was used, this intervention was accessible to employees with a range of literacy skills, including low literacy.

**Brug *et al.*, 1996 (3093) investigated a nutrition education intervention in a randomised trial involving 347 employees of a major oil company in The Netherlands. The intervention was based on the assumption that nutrition information tailored to the individual's characteristics, as provided by health counsellors for example, might be more effective than generalised nutrition education. Providing personalised nutrition education to a large population, however, is generally very expensive, but the use of computers may make it more feasible. The investigators developed a computerised system in which a total of 223 feedback messages written by professional health educators and a nutritionist, could be combined to more than 1 million different letters tailored to an individual's dietary intake of fat, fruit and vegetables and his/her psycho-social determinants of dietary intake.

A self-administered questionnaire assessed each individual's attitudes, social influences, self-efficacy and consumption levels which were then entered into the computer. The tailoring device was a collection of 'if–then' statements controlling the selection of feedback messages based on the screening results. The relevant feedback messages were put in a logical order in an easily readable personal letter sent to participants 2 to 3 weeks after completing the screening. The targeted outcomes were assessed again at 1-month follow-up and compared to the results in a comparison group which had completed the screening and received a letter in the same format as the experimental group but with general nutrition information based on leaflets and recommendations from the Netherlands Bureau for Food and Nutrition Education.

Reviewers concluded that this intervention was effective in changing fat consumption only, not fruit or vegetable consumption, by participants receiving tailored messages. It did not change their perceived social influence (i.e. dietary habits of important others including spouse, other members of the household, colleagues) or expectancy of social support from these 'important others'. Since the response rate at baseline was relatively high (74%) and a high proportion of the study population were men, the authors suggested that men are interested in nutrition information, at least when provided personally and tailored to their needs. Additional reasons for relatively high participation could be: the way the programme was presented (the study was presented as a collaboration between the company's health department and the University of Limburg) and the support of the company; and/or the relatively highly-educated population. Though initial participation was high, more than 30% dropped out of the study before the post-test. However, the authors indicated that there were no significant differences with those remaining in the study.

In the concurrent process evaluation, more people in the tailored-feedback group reported having read the letter completely, to have saved it and discussed it with others. This group also reported more often that the letter was of personal relevance, was specifically written for them, contained a lot of new information, was interesting, and was perceived to have increased their motivation to make changes in diet. No difference between the two groups was observed in ratings for comprehensibility and credibility of the letters. However, the tailored-feedback group were more positive about the appearance of their letter.

A cancer prevention and control intervention was implemented in 114 worksites and involved 111 worksites (28 000 employees) in its evaluation. It is the largest trial of its kind in the USA to date and is known as the Working Well Trial (**Sorensen et al., 1996 (3135)). The intervention was coordinated by four centres, which all targeted eating patterns, and three also targeted smoking and occupational exposure to carcinogens. One study centre that dealt with worksites where a smoking ban was in operation did not include smoking or carcinogen exposure, though it did include a focus on cancer screening practices. The common intervention protocol focused on: building awareness; action and skills training; and maintenance of behaviour and prevention of relapse. It was multi-level in its approach, i.e. involving individual, community, and organisational levels. Working groups were formed to develop specific intervention strategies based on the core concepts (see also 'Healthy alliances'). Interventions at the individual level included a kick-off event, interactive activities, posters and brochures, self-assessments, self-help materials, campaigns and contests and education through classes and groups. These interventions had three main goals: to increase motivation to change through increased awareness; to provide skills training for individuals ready to take action; and to maintain change through supportive changes at the organisational level. The latter included: a management assessment of current corporate policies, practices and environments with the aim of identifying potential barriers to health promotion and of raising awareness of upper-management to the need for policy review; development of plans to accelerate change in physical environment (for example, point-of-purchase food labelling of cafeteria/vending machines) through negotiation, consensus-building and conflict resolution; and the institutionalisation of change in order to change norms in the workplace. The control group consisted of sites where there was no intervention or an optional minimal intervention, for example, the distribution of printed materials such as posters and newsletters.

At 1-year follow-up, the authors concluded that there were significant increases in vegetable consumption and reductions in fat consumption, but not in smoking. The concurrent process evaluation indicated that there was a higher delivery of nutrition-focused interventions in three of the four study centres; and that participants were more likely to report awareness of nutrition than smoking. The authors suggested that these observations may provide an explanation for the observed positive changes in nutrition variables and the *status quo* in smoking behaviour. However, the reviewers judged the intervention to be ineffective as similar changes in nutrition outcomes occurred in the control group.

Using results from a needs assessment and focus groups, a 6-week lunchtime nutrition promotion programme was developed and tested with a predominantly white-collar population on a Canadian university campus (**Sheeshka and Woolcott, 1994 (3148)). The programme focused on the relationship between diet and body weight, cancer, heart disease, and osteoporosis, and used Canada's Guidelines for Healthy Eating to promote foods high in complex carbohydrates and low in fat. Programme components included: weekly presentations; computerised diet analyses; supermarket tours; take-home activities; and group walks. The multiple components of the intervention, together with personnel and financial constraints made it necessary to limit the intervention to a small number of people, i.e. those aged 40 years and over who had expressed an interest in a nutrition programme.

The intervention was considered to be effective for improving perceptions that healthful foods are costly, unpalatable, or time-consuming to prepare (i.e. disincentives), and the ability to follow healthy eating practices consistent with a low fat, high fibre diet in situations of varying difficulty (i.e. self-efficacy). The intervention did not change intentions to adopt healthy eating or attitudes related to the value placed on good health and reduced risk of disease in the future (i.e. outcome value), or the likelihood that reducing fat or increasing fibre intakes would lead to positive health outcomes, such as lowered risk of heart disease (i.e. outcome expectancy).

Alcohol abuse

In 1989, the Minnesota Mining and Manufacturing (3M) company developed a comprehensive alcohol and drug abuse prevention programme using multiple and interactive strategies aimed at altering workplace culture and promoting employee 'ownership' of the programme (★★Stoltzfus and Benson, 1994 (3126)). The three core components of the programme were: (1) supervisory training programme; (2) an all-employee educational programme; and (3) a peer-helper programme. The 10-hour supervisory training was aimed at culture change, prevention and early intervention, and involved all managers and supervisors. The impact of alcohol and drug abuse on work performance was discussed as well as the 3M Drug and Alcohol Policy and the companion *Guidelines for supervisors.* Supervisors and other employees then discussed how to create a workplace free of alcohol and drug abuse, after which the supervisors were taught skills ranging from prevention to intervention in addressing a range of employee problems. The core educational programme was a 2-hour 'guideline setting' programme in which employees were challenged through an interactive process to look at their attitudes, behaviours and decisions regarding drug and alcohol use. They were also required to formulate personal guidelines with the aim of enabling those who choose to drink, to do so in a safe and responsible manner. They were taught how to express their concern to co-workers or others whom they perceived as abusing drugs and/or alcohol. The peer-helper programme focused on interpersonal skill development, helping skills, knowledge of resources, and referral skills. The local Employee Assistance professional provided consultation, leadership, and support to peer helpers.

The major programme components were delivered over 9 months during working hours. Some programme elements were continued afterwards (for example, peer-helper training) and several booster sessions were offered. There was an optional component to help working parents prevent drug and alcohol abuse by their children. Several other strategies were used to support the programme including posters, literature, articles in the company's newsletter, contests, and incentives.

Though the peer-helper training was an important component in the programme, only 14% of employees participated, whereas 82% of employees participated in the seminar on personal guideline setting. At 3 months follow-up, the intervention was judged effective for measures of alcohol use, i.e. frequency and volume; it also reduced drinking-and-driving; riding with a driver who is under the influence; the negative impact of alcohol use on work; and showed an improvement in a 10-item at-risk index. The intervention was ineffective for smoking and marijuana use, most likely due to the extremely low levels of use at pre-test. Sustained impact at 16 months follow-up as claimed by the authors, was judged by the reviewers as unclear due to the absence of data from the control group in which the intervention had been introduced in the meantime. The authors reported subsequent improvement in this delayed-intervention group in at-risk behaviour, negative impact of alcohol use on work, employee empowerment, and employee morale.

The authors indicated several factors as favourable to developing and delivering this intervention: strong management support; the involvement of an employee task force to coordinate and direct the effort; the positive emphasis on being responsible and caring about co-workers; the use of multiple strategies to communicate and repeat core messages; and linking the programme to existing plant safety, quality and productivity initiatives. The authors stated that plans were in process to refine and replicate the programme in 70 manufacturing sites over a 3-year period; and that a pilot study would be initiated at 3M's headquarters as well as with the sales force.

Another alcohol abuse prevention programme, the Working People Program, was field-tested with 108 predominantly blue-collar workers (**Cook, Back and Trudeau, 1996 (3143)). Its central elements were self-efficacy enhancement, improvement of social resistance skills, and bolstering of social support. The programme attempted to balance messages about the risks of alcohol misuse with messages about the benefits of healthy behaviours, and was delivered in four 30-minute sessions in company time over a period of 4 weeks. Each session included a video and a pamphlet with factual information, behavioural guidelines, and exercises and tools to aid in selecting and attempting healthy alternatives to substance misuse, presented in the context of a group discussion. Two work units from the main plant, each with approximately 260 employees, and all 95 employees from the branch facility were invited by mail to participate in an 'alcohol abuse' research programme. They were paid $5 if they filled out both the pre- and the post-test questionnaires.

The impact of the intervention was assessed immediately after the intervention and was found to be effective in changing motivation to reduce alcohol use, in decreasing the number of drinking days and heavy drinking. However, the programme was ineffective for self-efficacy for drinking reduction, health beliefs and stages of change, experiencing problems at work due to alcohol, and the average number of drinks consumed on drinking days. A low participation rate and a relatively high drop-out rate were major problems. More female employees remained in the study though the intervention was mainly targeted at male workers. Most of those remaining in the study rated the programme in general, and the videos and brochures in particular, as very good or excellent. The authors indicated that though the human resources director was supportive of the programme, the stance of the line management generally ranged from tolerance to resistance. Overt encouragement for participation was rare.

Osteoporosis

**Brown, 1996 (3089), reported on the effect of different delivery methods on the impact of four learn-at-home lessons about the prevention of osteoporosis. These lessons outlined the risk factors and the connection with dietary intake; emphasised control over certain risk factors; and suggested steps to reduce personal risk by eating calcium-rich foods, exercising regularly, and cautioning against the use of calcium supplements. Two methods of delivery were compared: impersonal delivery by the worksite coordinator, usually a personnel employee; and a group-delivery involving a 30-minute motivational meeting prior to distributing each lesson. This meeting included a short presentation of the main points of each lesson, emphasising the need for completion at home, a taste of a recipe using the food featured in the lesson, and a pep talk followed by a group vote to try out a specific activity, for example, trying a recipe; walking to establish regular exercise; involving the children in food preparation activities; and eating calcium-rich foods instead of supplements. The delivery approaches were adapted according to feedback from a sample of employed women and from intervention providers, indicating that short, direct interventions with minimal environmental support were preferred. The control group received learn-at-home lessons on cancer prevention delivered in an impersonal way. These lessons emphasised eating less fat and more vegetables, and practising self-examination for early signs of cancer.

Immediately after intervention, a significant increase in behaviour-habits score for both groups receiving the osteoporosis lessons was found, though only the group-delivery condition maintained a higher score at 4 months follow-up. The group-delivery approach, however, did not lead to significantly greater increases in calcium ratio than the impersonal delivery method. Both osteoporosis groups showed a significant gain in knowledge, with the group-delivery method scoring the highest gain. The attitudes and beliefs scores did not differ between groups at any time.

The attrition rate in this study was relatively high, ranging from 24% to 36% in different groups. However, the author provided data on those who dropped out of the study which indicated that they were significantly older, and those who dropped out of the experimental groups were more likely to be unmarried or to have younger children, and less likely to have a family history of osteoporosis. There were no significant differences in knowledge, attitudes or beliefs, but the non-completers in the group-delivery condition had a significantly better score for behaviour-habits at baseline. The reviewers concluded that the high attrition did not invalidate the author's conclusions on the effect of the intervention, but that caution has to be exercised in terms of the generalisability of the findings.

Healthy alliances

Several of the studies reviewed above involved potential recipients of the intervention in the development and/or delivery of the programme. In the study reported by **Erfurt, Foote and Heirich, 1991a (3024), all four sites hosting a wellness screening programme established a wellness coordinating committee that included representatives from management, labour and the plant medical department to help plan, coordinate, and carry out activities. The wellness coordinating committees were also involved in the planning of special events to encourage employees to take advantage of the services offered. The intervention was considered effective for smoking and blood pressure control, but not for weight control. See also 'Cardiovascular screening and risk assessment'.

**Parkinson et al., 1989 (3030), described the implementation and evaluation of the Coke Oven Intervention Program for reducing occupational cancer. The intervention was developed jointly by the United Steel Workers of America and the University of Pittsburgh. Health education sessions gave an overview of health and safety conditions; occupational cancer surveillance; regulations for personal practice in the workplace and engineering controls; and the current state of control at each plant. From the 28 operating coke plants in the US and Canada in 1984, matchable pairs (on geographic location, workforce size and ethnic composition) were sought. Seven pairs were obtained and one plant in each pair was randomised to receive the education programme or not. Participants improved significantly in their knowledge of the Coke Oven Standard and in workplace behaviours, with those attending multiple programmes showing the greatest benefit. People in the control sites interviewed on six occasions throughout the 2-year period showed little improvement. Parkinson et al. (1989, p. 471) stated that :

> The effective implementation of the programme was dependent on the unique collaboration between the union and the university. This collaboration began eight years before the development of the intervention programme and provided a foundation for an integrated approach to its design, implementation and evaluation. Specifically, the collaboration affected the substance of the programme, the presentations, the development and operation of a publicity campaign, the design and content of the questionnaires and telephone interview schedules, and the hiring and training of laid-off coke oven

workers who served as telephone interviewers. All levels of the union were involved in the programme, including the international office, district officials, and individual local unions… [the] programme was unique in combining the expertise of coke oven workers themselves and university personnel, and allowed [them] to meet fully the criteria for developing health education programmes espoused by the American Public Health Association.

The Live For Life Program (**Wilbur, Hartwell and Piserchia, 1986 (3074)) process began with its acceptance and support by top management. The management board in each company was asked to make three commitments: to give financial resources; to recruit volunteers from middle- and upper-management levels to work closely with the Live For Life administrator in managing the project; and to be responsive to employees' requests for environmental improvements. Although the administrator had no authority for the day-to-day operations of the on-site programme, his/her consultation and marketing strategy with company leadership aimed to ensure that the process was properly planned, organised and implemented in a way that satisfied the health enhancement needs of the entire base. The volunteer leaders group executed a range of functions including: the development of yearly marketing plans, participation objectives, and budget requirements; the development and execution of strategies for achieving targets; recommendations for environmental improvements to encourage and support employee participation and lifestyle change; and the preparation of periodic reports on programme results. They also organised different task forces including a cross-section of employees, around key areas of health such as exercise, smoking cessation, stress management, weight control/nutrition, publicity and general health knowledge. See also 'Cardiovascular screening and risk assessment'.

The Carolina Healthstyle programme (**Kronenfeld et al., 1987 (3019)) was coordinated by a limited number of full-time project staff who helped establishing healthstyle committees in the different state agencies involved. The committee's role was to select activities of interest in different areas of lifestyle change which were led by health educators employed by the project. After one year, agencies moved into a maintenance phase in which they were encouraged to use internal resources and community resources to provide group programmes directly. However, project staff were still available for consultation and specialised training. For example, training days were organised several times a year to motivate continued participation, provide health-related information as well as tips on how to plan health promotion activities. See also 'Cardiovascular screening and risk assessment'.

Some challenges of developing healthy alliances and evaluating their effectiveness were faced by the Take Heart Project (**Glasgow et al.,

1994 (3007)). To launch the project, worksites were invited to send at least two representatives to a Take Heart breakfast at which the project staff were introduced and the project described. Following mailed information and a telephone call, researchers visited worksites that had expressed an interest in implementing the project and aimed to secure the support from the top management in terms of: allowing employees paid time-off to participate in assessments; providing representatives to serve on an employee steering committee; and assisting in publicising the programme to employees. Union involvement was encouraged from the outset and the union was asked to help promote the programme and to provide representatives to serve on the steering committee. This committee selected activities best suited to the worksite from a menu of brief health education and environmental change activities.

The effectiveness of the intervention was tested in a multi-site randomised controlled trial which involved 26 moderate-size worksites (i.e. 125–750 employees). Matched sites were randomised to either an early- or delayed-implementation group. Two years later, no differences between groups were found in smoking, fat intake or cholesterol levels. Although these findings were disappointing, the authors could draw on their concurrent process evaluation to explore possible reasons and make recommendations for developing healthy alliances (★★Glasgow *et al.*, 1995, p. 215 (3070)):

> In our efforts to allow maximum choice and tailoring within the confines of our menu approach, we may not have been sufficiently structured early in the programme. Some steering committees grasped the menu concept and progressed rapidly, but others were substantially delayed in implementing their first Take Heart events. Greater direction from the research centre early in the programme might have helped. Steering committee composition may be critical as well. We provided guidelines for composition and ensured that each committee had representation from diverse employee groups, including management and labour, men and women, smokers and non-smokers, and employees from all major departments. Nevertheless, there were large differences across worksites in the steering committees' level of activity. In the second round of Take Heart, we are emphasising that steering committee members should be willing to get involved, to promote the programme among co-workers, and to participate in events rather than just attend meetings. We did not encourage interaction among early intervention worksites because of concerns about independence of effects. In retrospect, this may have been a mistake because many sites later expressed interest in what others were doing. In our current intervention we are encouraging and facilitating more interaction between sites, including going to meetings and the publication of a Take Heart newsletter so that information can be shared.

The Working Well Trial (**Sorensen *et al.*, 1996 (3135)) was coordinated by four centres and had three structural levels: (1) a decision-making structure across study centres to establish and coordinate the common administrative intervention; (2) a management structure within each study centre to implement the intervention; and (3) an employee advisory board and a coordinator within each individual worksite to help tailor and implement the intervention. A participatory strategy was used at the community level for planning and implementation of the intervention. An employee from each worksite was appointed as the worksite coordinator and served as a gatekeeper. Employee advisory boards with 4 to 12 representative members (top and middle management, line supervisors, manual labourers, unions, etc.) were formed as a way of incorporating employee input and concerns. Smokers as well as non-smokers had to be represented on the board. The members were trained in the goals and content areas of the project, and in their roles and responsibilities, and were provided with basic information regarding smoking and nutrition. Abrams *et al.* (1994, p. 24) indicated that:

> Developing and implementing effective interventions with heavy reliance on worker participation is challenging and takes longer than anticipated; constraints arising from the realities of worksites required modification and flexibility in research design and intervention strategies. Economic hardship, lay-offs and change in management disrupted the intervention strategies. ()

See also 'Healthy eating' above.

4. Studies carried out in the UK

Despite the Health of the Nation's emphasis on promoting healthy workplaces, published reports of evaluated worksite health promotion interventions in the UK are rare. In this review, 68% (15) of the UK-based studies published since 1994, were reports of surveys, reviews and other types of descriptive studies; 14% (3) were outcome evaluations; and 9% (2) were descriptions of interventions or process evaluations. Combined with the studies identified in an earlier review (France-Dawson et al., 1994), there were five published UK-based outcome evaluation studies. They focused on: physical fitness in relation to mental and physical wellbeing (*Daley and Parfitt, 1996 (3144)); fitness in the context of cardiovascular disease (*Tregoning, Gent and Stephenson, 1990 (3005)); cholesterol level (*Elton et al., 1994 (3047)); smoking (*Amos, White and Elton, 1995 (3158)); and accidents in the workplace (*Cooper et al., 1994 (3140)). Four of these did not match our inclusion criteria for this review. Two evaluations employed a post-test design; two a pre- and post-test; and one was a randomised controlled trial None of the studies was judged to be methodologically sound, so caution has to be taken in drawing conclusions from them. We briefly describe all studies here with the aim of maximising learning from these rare examples within the British context.

*Daley and Parfitt, 1996 (3144), assessed the differences in mood states, physical wellbeing, job satisfaction and absenteeism between members of a corporate health and fitness club, non-members, and those on a waiting list to join the club. The authors stated that the rationale for the evaluation was the lack of evidence in the UK supporting worksite health promotion as compared to the US, and argued that different societal and working values make it difficult to apply outcomes from the American studies to the British context. The authors concluded that members of the fitness club had better scores for physical and psychological wellbeing, job satisfaction and absenteeism. However, the authors indicated that they were unable to infer causality due to the use of a non-experimental design.

*Tregoning, Gent and Stephenson, 1990 (3005), reported on the effect of fitness testing in the context of a wider health promotion programme on diet, exercise, alcohol use and smoking behaviour targeted at non-manual workers of a civic centre and manual workers of an electrical manufacturing firm. All workers were invited to attend for exercise testing on a specific day. Participants filled in a pre-test questionnaire and pulse and blood pressure were measured together with grip strength and suppleness, body fat and aerobic exercise testing. At the end of this session, appropriate lifestyle advice was offered. The post-test questionnaire covered measures on diet, alcohol and physical exercise behaviours and data were compared between the non-manual and manual workers. The authors concluded that the health promotion programme was effective with greater benefits for manual workers as compared to non-manual workers. However, the study was effectively a post-test design only (the pre- and post-test questionnaires covered a different range of outcomes) with no control group, which invalidates the authors' conclusions.

*Elton *et al.*, 1994 (3047), conducted a randomised controlled trial to evaluate whether knowing one's serum cholesterol level had an effect on reducing cholesterol levels in chemical industry workers. All workers were invited to a health education session which lasted about an hour and advocated a standardised diet. Participants were handed a sealed envelope a quarter of an hour before the start of the session. For the intervention group, the envelope contained one of three different letters according to whether personal cholesterol level was higher or equal to 6.5 mmol/l ('high'), between 5.2 and 6.45 mmol/l ('not particularly high'), or 5.2 mmol/l or lower ('below average'). All letters indicated that the advice in the health education session should be followed irrespective of the cholesterol result, aiming to maintain or reduce serum cholesterol level as appropriate. The control group received a standard letter informing them that they were part of the control group but that the health education session was also relevant to them as it is worthwhile for everybody to reduce their cholesterol concentration. The authors were cautious in concluding that the intervention was effective – there was only a significant reduction in the serum cholesterol level of those whose initial concentration was 'high'. However, the reviewers judged the intervention as unclear in its effect because the evaluation was judged to be flawed in that pre- and post-intervention data were reported only for those remaining in the study. Also, the information on the randomisation procedure for this trial was unclear.

*Amos, White and Elton, 1995 (3158) evaluated a telephone helpline for smokers using a pre- and post-test design. After the implementation of a smoking ban, a telephone helpline was set up for all employees of British Telecom (BT) in response to a survey indicating that 44% of smokers would consider giving up smoking if information and advice were offered. The helpline provided information and advice on the no-smoking policy and offered additional services to smokers who wanted help giving-up. The latter included a literature pack containing leaflets and information about smoking and ways of quitting, a health check with the occupational health service and the opportunity to attend a presentation on smoking cessation at their workplace. Self-reported smoking behaviour data were collected from all employees who called the helpline during a 3-month period (January–March 1993). Callers were asked about their previous smoking history and were sent a questionnaire 3 months later. Over half the smokers (62%) who called the helpline reported having tried to stop smoking and 28% of these claimed they were still successful at 3 months follow-up. Process measures regarding the acceptability of the intervention indicated that callers evaluated the service positively with over two-thirds indicating that they were very or quite satisfied with the helpline and 58% indicating that the helpline or the additional services offered would be useful in helping them quit. Although careful not to claim effectiveness, the authors concluded that the helpline was an effective mechanism for a nationwide company to identify smokers wanting support in quitting and that it was a useful means of centrally administering support services.

Only one study met the inclusion criteria set for this review – it was the only published study to state that it was based on a needs assessment and to have involved employees in both the design and the implementation of the intervention. *Cooper *et al.*, 1994 (3140), evaluated an intervention which used a behavioural approach to reducing accidents in a large production plant using a pre- and post-test design. The intervention was designed in response to information from the safety committees of the worksite reporting that despite the fact that a number of strategies had been implemented to reduce accidents, there was still a base level of accidents which was difficult to reduce. Senior site management consulted employees who indicated that the majority of accidents were caused by individual behaviour. Therefore, the intervention focused on unsafe behaviours.

The intervention consisted of four components: observation of safety behaviours; feedback and goal setting; continuing feedback; and managerial support. Forty-eight employees were trained by researchers to observe their colleagues' safety performance and to complete checklists of critical behaviours within the worksite. Initial departmental goal-setting meetings were led by the researchers and the trained observers, where the purpose and the philosophy of the behavioural approach to reducing accidents in the workplace was explained. It was emphasised that no individual employee could be singled out and that no disciplinary action would be taken against individuals who did not follow the procedures advocated on the checklist. Within these meetings, the results of the baseline observations were presented in terms of the percentage of safe behaviour observed over the 4-week period. In order to promote workers' ownership of the project, they were divided into groups, each of which agreed on a particular goal in safety improvement that was difficult to obtain but nonetheless achievable. Subsequently, the group goals were averaged to provide the departmental goal. The latter was then used as a reference on the feedback charts on which results of observations were posted on a weekly basis. Managerial support was actively promoted and managers were asked to praise workers for safe behaviour. Senior management, including the chief executive, were asked to visit each department on a weekly basis to discuss and make comments on the progress made. Although the authors claimed an increase in safety behaviours and a decrease in accidents over the study period, reliable conclusions about the effectiveness of the intervention cannot be drawn because of the lack of a control group.

5. Discussion

Since there is a dearth of published UK-based studies on workplace health promotion, the discussion will mainly draw on studies conducted in the USA. However, most of the issues raised are of relevance to workplace health promotion in the UK.

The purpose of workplace health promotion

The main reason for providing health promotion interventions in the workplace is to address health needs identified by epidemiological data, rather than by the recipients themselves. In our review, 40% of included outcome evaluation studies stated they were exclusively based on 'normative' need (using an 'expert' definition of need), whereas only 14% stated they were exclusively based on 'felt' need (what people say they want or what they think are the problems that need addressing).

Though epidemiological need may be the main rationale, the provision of health promotion programmes does not always match this need. For example, a Canadian study examined lifestyle indicators and the prevalence of interventions across work sectors (MacDonald and Wells, 1995). The study found that people in service-, construction- and trade-work sectors had a higher proportion of lifestyle problems (alcohol consumption, smoking, and stress) than those in health, education and government sectors, but that programmes addressing these issues were most prevalent in primary resources, government and health sectors and least prevalent in construction, trade and transportation.

Corporations have a vested interest in health if for no other reason than to eliminate excess costs in their products and services; according to the US Health Care Financing Administration, companies are currently spending 48% of their after tax profits on the provision of medical care for their employees and dependents (Pelletier, 1993). But, from the perspective of the health community, one hopes that the principal economic concern will shift from the intervention's ability to save money to its ability to improve employee health in a cost-effective way (Pelletier, 1991). As UK-employers increasingly offer private health insurance schemes to a wide range of employees, the economic benefits of workplace health promotion experienced in North America become more relevant to the UK. Currently, extrapolation of the effects on productivity, absenteeism, morale and company image from the US to the UK may be more relevant (Sanders and Crowe, 1996).

The number of organisations offering health promotion programmes at the worksite has grown exponentially since 1980 in the USA, with 81% of worksites offering some type of programme for their employees (Wilson, Holman and Hammock, 1996). While employers may endorse occupational health in principle, few transfer this support into practice in the UK. Surveys of public and private sector employers and trade unions in the UK have shown that health promotion programmes are receiving increasing attention, although they are by no means universal (Sanders and Crowe, 1996; Springett and Dugdill, 1995). Sadler and Thomas (1994) report on the Wellbeing at Work initiative set up by Birmingham City Council focusing on the needs of companies and social inequalities in health. The researchers found that few of the 150 firms surveyed provided an occupational health service for their employees even though the majority were convinced that the provision of an occupational health service reduces sickness absence. A survey of a representative sample of 1344 workplaces in England indicated that 40% undertook at least one major health-related activity in the previous year (HEA, 1993), but it is the larger companies that engage most in such activities (Springett and Dugdill, 1995). Sanders and Crowe (1996) caution that although encouraging, these findings may be an overestimate due to response bias: companies which have an interest in health promotion may be more likely to respond to surveys than those with little interest and little or no activity. Since there is no legal requirement for occupational health services except in dangerous occupations, and little development of a coordinated occupational health service in the National Health Service, health promotion programmes have tended to be adopted on an *ad hoc* basis with very little systematic evaluation (Sanders and Crowe, 1996). However, persuading companies to invest in health promotion has become easier, but persuading them to implement relevant programmes, in the appropriate way and to evaluate them properly has proved more difficult (Springett and Dugdill, 1995). Springett and Dugdill (1995) indicate the lack of financial and human resources, as well as time constraints as the main barriers to effective evaluation, especially for small and medium-sized enterprises. An enduring challenge is indeed the provision of occupational health services in smaller workplaces with relatively large fixed overhead costs per employee (Donaldson and Blanchard, 1995; Hagard, 1994), and the provision of health promotion programmes during periods of down-sizing and health care reforms (Wilson, Holman and Hammock, 1996).

According to Wilson, Holman and Hammock (1996) workplace health promotion has gone through an evolution: first generation programmes were offered for a number of reasons, most unrelated to health; second generation programmes were characterised by a focus on a single intervention or behaviour and targeted toward one population; third generation programmes were designed to offer a variety of interventions aimed at a variety of risk factors or behaviours for all employees; and, finally, fourth generation programmes encompassed a comprehensive approach incorporating all activities, policies, and decisions related to the health of employees, their families, the communities in which they reside, and the company's consumers. The comprehensive approach has taken a variety of forms but generally reflects both individual, organisational and community levels of change. Wilson, Holman and Hammock (1996) suggest that, at the individual level, the cornerstone of any health promotion effort is a well-designed employee education programme which may be conducted in a variety of formats using a multitude of strategies. At the organisational level, support mechanisms are required throughout the organisation to reinforce and encourage positive health actions; these should include formal policies backed by the organisational structure, including managers and supervisors. Finally, at the community level, efforts to educate and provide support mechanisms for the family and community are important, not just in an attempt to affect health care costs, but also on the grounds that these groups affect 'off-duty' behaviour and ultimately compromise the organisation's future workforce (Wilson, Holman and Hammock, 1996).

The evidence for workplace health promotion

Our review findings resonate with those of other recently conducted reviews of workplace health promotion (Anderson and Staufacker, 1996; Dugdill and Springett, 1994; Glanz, Sorensen and Farmer, 1996; Hennrikus and Jeffery, 1996; Roman and Blum, 1996; Shephard, 1996; Wilson, Holman and Hammock, 1996; Wilson, Jorgensen and Cole, 1996). General conclusions are that:

- most interventions are targeted at the individual level, though some are supported by environmental modifications of a varying degree;

- the relative effectiveness of specific intervention approaches is unclear;

- long-term effects have yet to be demonstrated;

- the quality of worksite research and evaluation should be significantly enhanced so that more studies use strong research designs including randomisation, replication across sites, consistent documentation, investigation of a range of outcomes, and improved characterisation of organisational factors that might be related to success.

As other authors of systematic reviews have stated, the rating for the quality of evidence in the literature as a whole lies between suggestive and indicative. Conclusive evidence about a causal relationship between worksite health promotion and improved behaviour or health is not yet available, but impact is plausible (Glanz, Sorensen and Farmer, 1996; Wilson, Jorgensen and Cole, 1996).

Although data supporting worksite programmes are not definitive, health promotion and disease prevention research is improving, and one of the outcomes will be to realise how deficient some of the earlier studies may have been. Virtually all worksite programmes to date have been focused on primary prevention, but as both interventions and evaluations move into secondary and tertiary prevention areas, it will be increasingly possible to prove or disprove both health and cost benefits, given the more evident benefits and higher costs associated with higher-risk and/or ill populations served by secondary and tertiary prevention programmes (Pelletier, 1993). Stokols, Pelletier and Fielding (1995) call for evaluations that consolidate previously disparate measures of the health impacts of worksite interventions: biomedical, behavioural, and psychological indices of employee health. A priority should be the development of improved methods for evaluating the financial and organisational outcomes of interventions and the incorporation of a wider array of productivity and organisational effectiveness criteria such as: quantity, quality and timeliness of employees' work performance; aggregate rates of absenteeism; staff turnover and retention; frequency and quality of communication among co-workers; and the company's reputation in the broader community (Stokols, Pelletier and Fielding, 1995).

Workplace health promotion programmes ideally should not only focus on individual behaviour and threats arising from the chemical, physical and biological environments, but should also include a focus on the 'newly recognised threats to health' arising from the psycho-social environment (Karasek and Theorell, 1990; Springett and Dugdill, 1995). Springett and Dugdill (1995) indicate a need for a more comprehensive, holistic approach to the evaluation of such programmes and the development of new research paradigms such as action research, and validated evaluation tools to measure both health needs and health gains. They expect such approaches to be more successful in addressing the real health needs of the working population and therefore those individuals who are least likely to participate in health promotion programmes (Springett and Dugdill, 1995).

An increasingly common theme among evaluators regardless of their epistemological orientation, is that multiple methods should be used in programme evaluation, as they increase the validity of the conclusions and the range of information collected (Israel *et al.,* 1995). Ideally most evaluations should include sufficient quantitative data to be able to assess the reach and generalisability of an intervention, and qualitative data to determine the depth and significance of change for individuals and communities, including any unintended effects. Clark and McLeroy (1995) indicate the need for ways to bring together more effectively both quantitative and qualitative approaches.

Participation in workplace health promotion

Because the public health significance of worksite interventions depends on the interest and willingness of employers to support such programmes and of employees to participate, an important aspect is how to make them more attractive.

In our review, the participation rate varied from 2% to nearly 100%, with most studies (42%) not stating their participation rate, 34% reported a participation rate of over 50% and 18% reported participation to be below 50%; 6% were unclear. Participation, however, can be defined very broadly to include any programme activity, with the consequence that the amount and intensity of activity probably varies substantially among employees which may affect the results (Fielding *et al.*, 1995).

Only 3 (6%) studies had non-voluntary participation. The Minnesota Mining and Manufacturing company's alcohol and drug prevention programme was based on the operational principle that mandated participation by all employees, and that management would demonstrate commitment to and investment in the programme. Eighty-four per cent supported the programme at pre-test and 64% advocated introducing the programme at other worksites (★★Stoltzfus and Benson, 1994 (3126)). In another study, the general maintenance workers at a university campus involved in a daily morning stretch and exercise programme to reduce injuries, sick leave and compensation claims, initially expressed resentment over the mandatory participation. However, a survey later on in the programme indicated general support for the programme and enthusiasm for continuation. The authors indicated that exercising as a group reinforced people's willingness to participate and promoted a team feeling (★Davis and Johnson, 1994 (3137)). The study reported by Cooper *et al.* (1994 (3140)) involved all employees, including the management of a manufacturing plant. Though all employees were being observed for their safety behaviours by trained peers, they were assured that no one individual could be identified and that no disciplinary action would be taken against those not following the recommended procedures.

Several studies have reported on the effect of social factors such as class, gender, ethnicity and employee status on participation rate. People who elect to participate are more likely to be older, more educated, white collar workers, already committed to healthy lifestyles (Carter *et al.,* 1995; Cirksena and Flora, 1995; Lerman and Shemer, 1996; Lusk, Kerr and Ronis, 1995). They may be more highly motivated and may thus improve their health regardless of programme participation. One can thus assume that those who need the programmes least are most likely to participate (Sepulveda, Goetz and Grana, 1994).

Emmons *et al.* (1996) and Sorensen *et al.* (1996) carried out studies on participation in the context of the Working Well Trial (**Sorensen *et al.,* 1996 (3135)). Emmons *et al.* (1996) investigated the barriers to women's participation. They found that low-risk non-participants (low risk was defined as: not smoking, exercising at least 20 minutes three times a week, obtaining less than 30% of calories from fat) wanted to take personal responsibility for their health and were already participating in health promotion activities outside the workplace. Moderate-risk and high-risk non-participants focused on past failures, were suspicious regarding the motives for health promotion, and viewed the work environment as non-supportive. A common barrier to participation regardless of risk status was lack of time. The authors therefore suggested that the limited resources should be focused on those subgroups who do not already participate in health promotion activities elsewhere; that attempts to minimise the stress and guilt surrounding health behaviours should be made; and that organisational changes should be incorporated to create a supportive environment. Sorensen *et al.* (1996) found that when workers were aware of changes their employers had made to reduce occupational hazards, they were more likely to participate in health promotion activities. They recommended a 'bargaining' approach, taking into account workers' more immediate health concerns, which involves visible management-led organisational changes that in turn could lead to enhanced participation in programmes aimed at individual behaviour change.

All of these findings suggest that the effort invested in planning workplace health promotion should be more responsive to the needs of workers as this could increase the potential of successful outcomes. Interventions should also take into account people's health behaviour practices as well as their definitions of health.

Developing feasible and acceptable interventions

Several of the studies included in our review involved the target/study population in the development and delivery of interventions. These have been discussed in 'Healthy alliances' in Chapter 3. There is no doubt that participatory methods improve the feasibility and acceptability of interventions. The extent to which these modify the participation rates and the impact of interventions is currently not clear.

A good example of how focus group interviews with a sample of the study population considerably modified the programme content of an alcohol intervention, is reported in the study by *Kishchuk et al., 1994 (3091). Messages on weekly safe drinking limits made little sense as participants reported that drinks were all likely to be consumed during the same evening. The weekly limits were eliminated from the programme, only per-occasion limits were retained. All of the elements derived from the clinical literature on controlled consumption were judged unacceptable. Participants felt insulted by any suggestions that they should manage or control their drinking, as this was equated with having a drinking problem. The 'drinking diaries', which are often a feature of programmes for problem drinkers, were judged particularly objectionable. These elements were also eliminated from the intervention, except for a brief mention of several hints for avoiding undesired levels of intoxication such as alternating non-alcoholic with alcohol beverages. Participants further indicated the parts of the programme they would like to see expanded such as information on statistics about the social cost of alcohol, and training on how to diplomatically but effectively intervene with a family member or friend who had had too much to drink. Several elements promoting self-efficacy in drinking management were therefore included. The reviewers judged this intervention as unclear in its effect, since the groups included in the evaluation were not equivalent in socio-demographic characteristics and information on pre-intervention outcome measures was not provided for all individuals.

While employment has a major influence on general wellbeing, health promotion activities in the workplace artificially separate work from other aspects of people's lives, which may have a particular effect on women whose specific needs, arising from the demands of their multiple roles, are often overlooked (Springett and Dugdill, 1995). Though a health needs assessment as the basis for determining the nature of an intervention is beginning to be seen as good practice, conventional approaches to needs assessment still tend to reinforce the view that health is about individual lifestyle only. Participatory approaches may overcome some of these problems and increase the likelihood that different experiences are articulated and subsequently incorporated in the agenda for change (Springett and Dugdill, 1995).

The role of health promotion providers

Several descriptive studies examine the role of, and relationships between, providers of health promotion in and outside the workplace, including occupational nurses, physicians, other primary health care staff and employers. The main debate concerns the merits of occupational health and of health promotion and how they can complement one another (see Blewett and Shaw, 1995). Kogan (1996) argues that occupational health physicians might be spreading themselves too thinly by adopting health screening and education initiatives, and stresses the importance of the profession's priority, i.e. protecting employees from the hazards of work. Heaney and Goldenhar (1996), however, argue for the integration of workplace health promotion and occupational health and safety to advance the quality and scope of worksite health programmes.

Parker (1996) surveyed 400 British general practitioners (GPs) and occupational physicians about their attitudes to workplace health services. Though there was support for the usefulness of workplace health promotion, there was a lack of consensus among the professionals to provide specific health screening and vaccination at work. Several GPs expressed concern about workplace screening tests for cardiovascular risk factors or vaccinations, if the patients subsequently had to be followed-up for problems and adverse reactions. Few GPs acknowledged the opportunity for alcohol counselling in the workplace. Parker highlights the need for more effective communication between occupational physicians and GPs; for an increase in GPs' knowledge of occupational medicine; and an increase in professional links between the specialities in order to avoid duplication of effort.

There is a growing trend in the provision of occupational health and safety services to consider cost-effectiveness. A review of the training of occupational physicians in Britain (Deacon 1996) recommended the inclusion of strategic business appraisal, organisational planning and accountancy, and risk assessment training. Other aspects of planning and evaluation for occupational health programmes should include: customer need; costs; quality; and audit. Occupational physicians need to appreciate the benefits of using the same management tools as employers.

Though the above mentioned studies seem to be limited to health professionals as providers of health promotion programmes in the worksite, our review identified some outcome evaluations of interventions that have involved a range of providers: community and social workers; counsellors and psychologists; health professionals; health promotion practitioners; and peers. In fact, only one sound and effective study was identified in which a health professional (a medical consultant) was involved – the United Steel Workers of America coke oven intervention programme, extensively described above (★★Parkinson et al., 1989 (3030)). This is not necessarily a reflection on the ability of health professionals to provide effective health promotion interventions, but rather on the overall quality of evaluation studies.

Appendices

Appendix A. Evaluating interventions and defining and measuring outcomes

Evaluation can be defined as the determination of the effectiveness, efficiency and acceptability of a planned intervention in achieving stated objectives (Homans and Aggleton, 1989). The requirements of adequate intervention development, implementation and evaluation have been described by Zaslow and Takanishi (1993) as follows:

1. a descriptive (qualitative) phase of understanding the norms and range of behaviours of the target group;

2. based on these data, the development of specific hypotheses and theories about why such behaviour occurs;

3. the design and implementation of theory-driven intervention strategies;

4. full documentation of the programme;

5. evaluation of its short-term impact by using random assignment to groups and proven behavioural outcome measures conceptually related to the hypotheses under test;

6. distinguishing short-term effects;

7. trying to describe underlying processes;

8. longitudinal studies to determine the extent to which the effects are sustained over time.

The term 'evaluation' covers studies which aim to describe both *processes* and *outcomes* (Coyle, Boruch and Turner, 1991). *Process* evaluations study the ways in which services or interventions are delivered. They are designed to describe what goes on rather than to establish whether it works or not. *Outcome* evaluations are designed in such a way that they can generate answers to questions about the effectiveness of particular interventions in changing specified outcomes. Many evaluations claiming to provide data on outcomes are really exercises in monitoring or surveillance. They make claims about the effects of interventions rather than establishing effectiveness.

Randomised controlled trials (RCTs) provide a remedy to the inferential uncertainties of non-experimental designs. They offer a means of establishing the effectiveness of different approaches to a problem, largely through securing an equivalence between the social characteristics of experimental and control groups, distributing unknown factors capable of influencing outcome equally between study groups, and reducing the possibility of researcher bias (Chalmers, Enkin and Keirse, 1989; Chalmers *et al.*, 1983; Schwartz, Flamant and Lellouch, 1980; Silverman, 1985). This offers the best chance of any post-intervention outcome differences between the randomly selected groups being due to the effects of the intervention itself.

The primary condition for a RCT is uncertainty about the effectiveness of a particular intervention. If there is certainty, based on sound scientific evidence, then a RCT is both unnecessary and unethical. In the face of *un*certainty, a RCT is ethical, and, by extension, any other approach to assessing effectiveness which cannot, for design reasons, be expected to generate an answer becomes *un*ethical. However, what is ethical may not be considered possible for practical or political reasons.

There is a widespread debate within the health promotion and general academic communities about the relevance of RCTs to the evaluation of social interventions, and this is not the place to repeat this debate (but see for example, Oakley and Fullerton, 1996; Oakley, 1998; Speller, Learmonth and Harrison, 1997). Much of the debate is concerned with questions other than effectiveness and some is based on a misunderstanding of the design of RCTs as 'socially equitable comparison tests'. The premise on which the review described in this report is based, is that the rationale for most workplace health promotion is the possibility of reducing health-risk behaviours, and the most efficient way to evaluate effectiveness is to use a strong design which enables the programme's impact to be assessed against the standard of outcomes in a 'no intervention' control population.

There can be many different measures of the outcomes of health promotion programmes aimed at employed people. These range from knowledge, awareness, attitudes and self-efficacy to skill development, reported behaviour and clinical risk factors or health status. Most health promotion interventions do not aim to influence the whole range of possible outcomes. Some reports of evaluations are unclear about the range of outcomes targeted, and/or they describe a broad list of aims which are not matched with appropriate outcome measures and/or they fail to report data for all outcomes targeted.

Appendix B. Methodology of the review

This review involved the following stages of work:

1. Using literature searches to identify studies in the area of interest.

2. Collecting full reports of relevant studies.

3. Classifying reports according to study design, country, health area, study population and, in the case of intervention studies, also for the type of intervention and the intervention provider, by means of a standardised coding strategy.

4. Assessing the evaluation studies for the presence of inclusion criteria.

5. Compiling on to a specialised computer database, EPIC, information on the planning, content, delivery and implementation of the intervention, the study population and the evaluation design of included studies.

6. Assessing the methodological quality of the evaluations in order to identify the subset from which potentially reliable conclusions can be drawn.

7. Generating descriptions of the field of interest from all studies and conclusions on the effectiveness of interventions from the subset of reliable studies using EPIC.

Identification and classification of relevant studies

We developed search strategies with a high sensitivity for identifying outcome evaluations of health promotion interventions in the workplace (see Appendix C). Search results were scanned and all workplace health promotion-related studies were coded, using a standardised coding strategy developed by the EPI-Centre for the type of study, the country where the study was carried out, the health focus, the study population and, in case of intervention studies, also for the type of intervention and the intervention provider. The search results were subsequently entered into BiblioMap, the EPI-Centre register of health promotion studies.

Inclusion/exclusion criteria

The focus was on risk-reduction behaviours relevant to the prevention of disease and the promotion of healthy lifestyles. Evaluation studies were included if they tested interventions aimed either directly (at the individual level) or indirectly (at the organisational level) at behaviour change. Interventions which involved improving elements in the biological, physical or chemical workplace environment with no implications for behaviour change were excluded.

All relevant outcome evaluations for which the full report could be obtained within the time limit set for the review were screened according to the following inclusion/exclusion criteria:

1. Whether the evaluation had been carried out retrospectively or prospectively

To maximise the validity of the review conclusions, retrospective studies were excluded.

2. Whether smoking prevention/cessation was the main focus of the intervention

Evaluation studies exclusively focusing on smoking were excluded to avoid duplication of effort with the Cochrane Review Group on Tobacco Control. Details of completed and continuing systematic reviews of the effectiveness of different smoking prevention/cessation interventions are available on the Cochrane Library database (Cochrane Library, 1998).

In addition, a study had to meet *at least one* of the following inclusion criteria :

3. Development of the intervention on the basis of a needs assessment and/or participatory methods

For health promotion interventions to be both necessary and relevant, they should be based on a needs assessment and developed by involving the people for whom they are intended. At the very least, programmes should be piloted and their content and delivery amended according to the participants' views, before an extensive outcome evaluation is undertaken.

We restricted the inclusion of studies to outcome evaluations of interventions that were based on a needs assessment and/or developed using participatory methods and/or previously piloted with the study/target population. Evaluation reports of interventions exclusively based on 'normative' need (using an 'expert' definition of need) were excluded, as were those reporting on interventions that were previously piloted but did not provide any further details of how the pilot findings were dealt with.

4. The inclusion of process as well as outcome measures

To maximise learning from this review, we limited inclusion to outcome evaluations which included at least one process measure other than programme reach or implementation monitoring.

These criteria were used with the aim of contributing towards the integration of qualitative and quantitative methods within effectiveness reviews.

Assessing methodological quality

Studies classified as outcome evaluations were reviewed for the presence/absence of eight methodological qualities, as follows:

1. Clear definition of the aims of the intervention

Critical to the measurement of effectiveness is the determination of relevant outcome measures as indicators of success. Many studies aim to assess the success of a given intervention on two or more outcomes, such as knowledge about specific health risks and behavioural changes, but report only the 'successful' outcome measures.

2. A description of the study design and content of the intervention sufficiently detailed to allow replication

If a programme is found to demonstrate the desired outcome, it is crucial to identify whether or not success can be repeated if implemented by others in different settings. In order for this to be achieved, the content and design of the study should be described in such a way as to allow replication.

3. Use of random allocation to the different groups including to the control or comparison group(s)

In assessing the effectiveness of an intervention, two basic questions need to be addressed: first, are changes evident in the outcome variable(s); and second, can they be attributed to the intervention? The use of randomised allocation to experimental and comparison/control groups increases the confidence with which observed differences in outcomes can be attributed to the programme under investigation. *Note:* Randomisation most likely, but not always, results in comparable groups (on socio-demographic and outcome variables) at baseline. Therefore, all trials including randomised controlled trials, are also assessed for the baseline equivalence of the different groups involved.

4. Provision of data on numbers of participants recruited to each condition

5. Provision of pre-intervention data for each group

An exception was made for those studies using the Solomon four-group design (Campbell and Stanley, 1963). In this design, intervention and control/comparison groups are further randomised to receive pre-intervention surveys or not. This means that the usual range of pre-intervention data is not available for half the participants in each group.

6. Provision of post-intervention data for each group

7. Attrition reported for each group

Giving information about the number of participants recruited to experimental and comparison/control groups, and providing relevant data on all participants in each group both prior and following the intervention, are basic requirements for evaluating the effectiveness of a programme. It is also necessary to monitor attrition rates within each group. Non-equivalent attrition, in which the characteristics of participants who drop out differ from those remaining, is a major threat to the external validity of the study. Researchers can test for this by comparing drop-outs with those remaining in the study on the pre-test measures of the dependent variable(s) and on demographic characteristics. If differences emerge, they can be controlled for using statistical techniques such as analysis of covariance. Without such monitoring and statistical control, the external validity of the study is reduced, and programme impact can only be generalised to a population similar to the participants who remained in the study. In addition, if differential attrition between groups occurs, the internal validity of the study is compromised and the conclusions rendered unclear.

8. Findings reported for each outcome measure indicated in the aims of the study

As noted above, a typical pattern is for reports of programme impact to include only outcome measures suggesting programme success, rather than outcome measures relating to all the pre-specified aims of the study.

A study displaying all of the attributes discussed above could be described as achieving a 'gold standard'.

Following on from other work (Fullerton and Oakley, 1995; Loevinsohn, 1990; MacDonald, Sheldon and Gillespie, 1992) a smaller group of 'core' criteria from the above list was selected in order to divide the studies into two broad groups: 'sound' and 'flawed'. 'Sound' studies were those deemed to meet at least the four criteria of:

1. employing a control/comparison group equivalent at baseline to the intervention group on socio-demographic and outcome variables;

2. providing pre-intervention data for each group;

3. providing post-intervention data for each group;

4. reporting on all outcomes targeted.

In view of the very small number of 'gold standard' studies the reviewing process identified, it was decided not to restrict 'sound' studies to those using randomised controls, but to include those where control/comparison groups/participants were demonstrated to be comparable to intervention groups/participants on socio-demographic and outcome variables. It was also decided to omit the criterion of replicability from the 'core' list on the grounds that interventions might potentially have been described in sufficient detail to be replicable, but that space limits in journals could have prevented this.

Two reviewers independently assessed each study; any disagreements were discussed and resolved with a third reviewer if necessary. A final element in the reviewing process consisted of judging the effectiveness of the programme from the information provided in the reports, and bearing in mind the 'quality' attributes referred to above. These reviewers' assessments of effectiveness were then contrasted with those provided by the authors themselves.

Note
As there were very few reports of UK-based outcome evaluation studies, we described all of them regardless of their match with the inclusion criteria or methodological criteria. They are discussed in Chapter 4. Caution has to be taken in drawing conclusions from these studies as none of the evaluations met the minimum quality criteria discussed above.

Appendix C. Identification of workplace health promotion reports

Search strategies

This review updates a review by Frances-Dawson *et al.* (1994) which included studies published up to early 1994. New reports of outcome evaluation studies published in the English language since 1994 were sought by systematic hand- and electronic database searches, through personal contacts, and by scanning the reference lists of reports of outcome evaluation studies.

The following journals and issues were hand-searched: *American Journal of Health Promotion* (January/February 1994 to January/February 1997); *American Journal of Public Health* (January 1994 to December 1996); *Health Education Quarterly* (Spring 1994 to November 1996); *Journal of Nutrition Education* (January/February 1994 to November/December 1996); *Journal of Occupational and Environmental Medicine*, previously known as *Journal of Occupational Medicine* until January 1995 (January 1994 to March 1997) and *Preventive Medicine* (January 1994 to January/February 1997).

Electronic searches covered: EMBASE; ERIC; Medline; PsycLIT and the Social Science Citation Index. Search strategies were developed for each of the databases. In all cases, searches were limited to the period 1994–1997.

1. EMBASE

The search strategy was developed by using appropriate EMTREE terms from the thesaurus.

Key

(expl):   searches for the chosen term and all its associated and subsidiary (explosion) terms.

(assoc): searches for the chosen term both as a major or as a minor term.

#1 *Health Education (expl)*
Health Promotion (assoc)
Patient Education (assoc)

#2 *Health Behavior (expl)*
Alcohol Abstinence (assoc)
Drinking Behavior (assoc)
Smoking Cessation (assoc)

#3 *Health Promotion (assoc)*

#4 *Primary Prevention (assoc)*

#5 *Work (expl)*
Work Environment (expl)
Absenteeism (assoc) personnel management (assoc)
Burnout (assoc) pneumatic tool (assoc)
Human factors research (assoc) trade union (assoc)
Job analysis (assoc) work capacity (assoc)
Job performance(assoc) work schedule (assoc)
Job satisfaction (assoc) working time (assoc)
Man machine interaction (assoc) work load (assoc)
Manual labour (assoc) work place(assoc)
Night work (assoc)
#7 (#1 or #2 or #3 or #4) AND (#5)

2. ERIC (Silver Platter)
Appropriate health-related terms from the thesaurus were combined
with relevant work-related terms from the index.
Key
explode: retrieves all references with the chosen term and its associated
narrower terms.
DE: searches for a term in the descriptive field of the record.

#1 *Health education* in DE

#2 *explode Health programs*
Breakfast programs
Immunization programs
Lunch programs
Mental health programs

#3 *Health promotion* in DE

#4 *Health related fitness* in DE

#5 *Occupational safety and health* in DE

#6 explode *Physical health*
Dental health
Physical fitness

#7 *Prevention* in DE
(includes Accident-prevention and Hearing-conservation in DE)

#8 *Preventive medicine* in DE

#9 *Workplace/worksite/workers* (from index)

#10 (#1 or #2 or #3 or #4 or #5 or #6 or #7 or #8) AND #9

3. Medline (Spirs)

MeSH headings were searched for using all subheadings and the explosion term when present.

#1 explode *Health-behaviour*/all subheadings

#2 explode *Health-education*/all subheadings

#3 *Health-promotion*/all subheadings

#4 explode *Primary-prevention*/all subheadings

#5 explode *Work*/all subheadings

#6 *Workplace*/all subheadings

#7 (#1 or #2 or #3 or #4) AND (#5 and #6)

4. PsycLIT (Spirs)

Relevant terms were chosen from the thesaurus. Since there were no descriptor phrases which referred to the workplace in the appropriate context, all terms from the index beginning with the word 'work' were selected.

#1 *Health-behavior* in DE

#2 explode *Health-care-psychology* in DE
Medical psychology

#3 explode *Health-education* in DE
Drug education
Sex education

#4 *Health-promotion* in DE

#5 *Prevention –* in DE

#6 *AIDS-prevention* in DE

#7 *Drug-abuse-prevention* in DE

#8 *Preventive-medicine* in DE

#9 *Primary-mental-health-prevention* in DE

#10 *Relapse-prevention* in DE

#11 explode *Health-screening* in DE
Cancer screening
HIV testing
Physical examination

#12 All index terms beginning with *'work'*

#13 (#1 or #2 or #3 or #4 or #5 or #6 or #7 or #8 or #9 or #10 or #11) AND #12

5. Social Science Citation Index (BIDS)
A free text search, using relevant terms in a truncated ($\star$) way, was used since no thesaurus or index is available.

#1 Health promotion

#2 Health education

#3 Health behavior$\star$

#4 Health behaviour$\star$

#5 Prevention

#6 Work-site$\star$

#7 Work-place$\star$

#8 Workplace$\star$

#9 Worksite$\star$

#10 (#1 or #2 or #3 or #4 or #5) AND (#6 or #7 or #8 or #9)

Search results
The searches carried out for the review by France-Dawson *et al.* (1994) identified 594 reports related to workplace health promotion of which 60 reported on separate outcome evaluation studies.

The literature searches carried out for this update identified a further 394 reports on workplace health promotion, 40% of which were located by two or more different methods of searching. Electronic database searching located 78% of the total relevant publications and 83% of the outcome evaluations. The largest proportion of both relevant reports (43%) and relevant outcome evaluations (41%) were identified from EMBASE. Medline identified 19% and 26% respectively; PsycLIT 15% and 18%; the Social Science Citation Index 20% and 15%; and ERIC identified the least number of relevant reports, 3% of all studies and 2% of outcome evaluations. Hand-searching located a substantial proportion of all relevant studies (36%) and outcome evaluations (41%); personal contact 4% and 5% respectively. Additional non-systematic scanning of bibliographies found 2% of all reports and 1% of outcome evaluations. (*Note*. Due to the overlap in studies identified by different methods percentages do not add to 100%.)

Of the 394 references, we were able to obtain 273 (69%) as full reports within the limited timeframe for the review, all of which were classified according to the type of study. For the citations for which full reports could not be obtained, classification was done on the basis of the information provided in the abstract (24% of all reports, 17% of outcome evaluations) or title (7% and 1% respectively). Table 1 summarises this information. Most (64%) of the papers reported descriptive studies; only 26% reported on outcome evaluations; and economic evaluations were rare (<1%).

Table 1: Framework for describing studies

	N	%
Total	394	100
Descriptive studies		
Survey	106	27
Review/Commentary	98	25
Systematic review/Meta-analysis	13	3
Case control/Cohort study	6	<2
Needs assessment	6	<2
Other	23	6
Intervention studies		
Non-evaluated intervention	27	7
Outcome evaluation only	76	19
Outcome and process evaluation	24	6
Process evaluation only	12	<3
Economic evaluation	3	<1

We were able to obtain 84 of the 100 outcome evaluations as full reports, these included two longer-term follow-up reports of outcome evaluations discussed in the review by France-Dawson *et al.* (1994). Hence, a total of 82 reports of separate outcome evaluations were newly identified for this update. Combined with the outcome evaluations identified in the earlier review (France-Dawson *et al.*, 1994), we assessed a total of 139 separate outcome evaluations for inclusion in this review.

Appendix D. Characteristics of the excluded versus included outcome evaluations

Of the 139 separate outcome evaluations (see Appendix C), 89 (64%) did not match the inclusion criteria: one was a retrospective study; 28 focused only on smoking; and 60 studies did not have at least one of the other required inclusion criteria set out in Appendix B. The majority of studies were published in 1990 or later (76% of excluded and 78% of included studies).

Table 2 compares the included and excluded outcome evaluation studies in terms of the country where the study was carried out, the focus and the type of intervention. Most studies were carried out in North America (81% of excluded and 94% of included studies); 4% or less were UK-based evaluations (representing a total of 5 studies).

Table 2: Included outcome evaluations (*N* = 50) versus excluded outcome evaluations (*N* = 89): percentage of studies displaying different characteristics in each group

	Included studies (%)	Excluded studies (%)
Country*		
North America	94	81
UK	<2	4
Other European	<2	7
Other	<4	8
Focus of the intervention†		
Alcohol abuse	16	1
Accidents	16	4
Cancer	16	6
Cardiovascular disease	28	24
Healthy eating	30	12
Mental health	20	16
Physical activity	24	19
Smoking	20	49
Weight loss	12	10
Other	18	11
Type of intervention†		
Advice/counselling	12	18
Environmental modification	22	8
Exercise	18	8
Increased access to resources/services	28	22
Information/education	84	56

Table 2: Included outcome evaluations (N = 50) versus excluded outcome evaluations (N = 89): percentage of studies displaying different characteristics in each group (cont'd)

	Included studies (%)	Excluded studies (%)
Type of intervention		
Legislation/regulation	6	18
Practical skill development	24	19
Risk assessment/screening	50	33
Social support	10	11
Other/Unclear	16	16

*Due to rounding up to the next whole figure, percentages do not add up to 100%.
†Some studies included more than one focus and/or type of intervention, thus percentages do not add up to 100%.

The majority of interventions targeted clinical risk factors (i.e. blood pressure, cholesterol level, weight) and/or behavioural risk factors (diet, exercise, smoking) for cardiovascular disease. Nearly all included an educational component (56% of excluded studies; 84% of included studies). Behavioural and/or clinical risk assessments, and/or medical screening were very common (33% and 50% respectively).

There were proportionally more interventions with a focus on alcohol, accidents, cancer, and healthy eating in the included studies. Environmental modification and exercise figured proportionally more often as a type of intervention in the included group, whereas interventions with a legislative/regulating component figured less often as compared to the excluded studies. The latter is mainly due to the exclusion of studies with a primary focus on smoking (49% of excluded studies), many of which evaluated smoking bans in the workplace. Overall, however, the range of interventions was fairly similar between the excluded and included studies, indicating that the inclusion criteria employed did not result in bias towards evaluations in a particular health area or of a particular intervention type.

Appendix E. Description of the included outcome evaluations

Fifty (36%) of the total of 139 separate outcome evaluations (see Appendix C) matched the inclusion criteria and were further assessed for methodological quality (see Appendix B). Only 15 (30%) of these were judged to be 'sound' evaluations from which potentially reliable conclusions can be drawn. Thirty-five (70%) were considered 'flawed' outcome evaluations. When referred to in the text, sound evaluations are starred twice ** and flawed evaluations once*.

Tables 3 and 4 give the basic data from the methodological review of the outcome evaluations. Nearly all the studies (90%) stated the aims of the intervention clearly; 32% were randomised controlled trials; 68% provided enough information to enable replication of both the intervention and the evaluation design; 88% gave the numbers recruited to each group in the study; 44% provided pre-intervention data for all groups; 52% included attrition rates and 60% reported post-intervention data for all groups; 82% of studies discussed the impact on all the outcomes specified as targets of the intervention (Table 3).

Table 3: Included outcome evaluations (N = 50): numbers/percentage of studies displaying different 'quality' criteria

	N	%
Aims clearly stated	45	90
Random allocation	16	32
Replicable intervention and evaluation design	34	68
Numbers recruited were provided	44	88
Pre-intervention data provided for each group	22	44
Attrition rates provided for each group	26	52
Post-intervention data provided for each group	30	60
The impact for all outcomes was discussed	41	82

Table 3 indicates that the main methodological problems of the reviewed studies were the failure to report pre- and/or post-intervention data as well as attrition rates for each group. This has serious implications for the interpretation of the findings from those studies.

Table 4 summarises the methodological data into the numbers of studies meeting the 8 'gold standard' methodological criteria and the four 'minimum standard' criteria (see Appendix B). Five studies (10%) met all eight quality criteria; 15 (30%) met the 4 minimum criteria. This group of 15 studies constituted our 'sound' group of studies from which potentially reliable conclusions on the effect of interventions can be drawn.

Table 4: Included outcome evaluations (*N* = 50): numbers/percentage of gold standard, sound and flawed evaluations

	N	%
Total*	50	100
Gold standard evaluations meeting all 8 methodological criteria	5	10
Sound evaluations meeting all 4 minimum standard criteria	15	30
Flawed evaluations NOT meeting all 4 minimum standard criteria	35	70

*Gold standard evaluations are also included in the group of sound evaluations, hence percentages do not add up to 50 or 100% respectively.

Part of our reviewing process consisted of comparing the claims to effectiveness made by authors of studies with those derived from the review process, bearing in mind the need for methodological soundness as a base for establishing effect. Tables 5 and 6 compare the effect of the interventions as judged from both these viewpoints.

Table 5 shows that most of the interventions, judged by the authors to be effective/ineffective/unclear in changing a range of outcome measures, were tested in evaluations that had some methodological flaws. This means that the authors' conclusions were unreliable for 70% of the interventions claimed effective, all of the interventions considered partially effective (i.e. effective for some groups only) or unclear; and 44% of the interventions considered ineffective for at least some of the targeted outcomes. Similarly, though none of the interventions were judged to be harmful, this may not necessarily be the case if tested by a rigorous evaluation design.

Table 5: Reliability of the authors' conclusions about the effect of interventions on a range of outcome measures

Authors' assessment of the *effect* of the intervention on different outcomes	Reviewers' assessment of the *quality* of the evaluation (N (%))		
	Sound	**Flawed***	**Total†**
Effective	13 (29%)	32 (71%)	45 (100%)
Effective – some groups only	0	5 (100%)	5 (100%)
Ineffective	9 (56%)	7 (44%)	16 (100%)
Unclear	0	2 (100%)	2 (100%)

*Conclusions about the effect of interventions cannot be drawn from flawed evaluations; the authors' conclusions in these cases are unreliable.

†Interventions targeted more than one outcome, hence numbers do not add up to 50 studies.

Table 6 shows that for all sound outcome evaluations (i.e. those from which potentially reliable conclusions can be drawn), the authors and reviewers did not necessarily agree on the impact of the intervention on the range of targeted outcomes. There was 73% agreement between authors and reviewers on the positive effect of the intervention on some of the targeted outcomes. They also agreed that in 60% of the cases the interventions had no impact on other targeted outcomes (i.e. were ineffective). In 66% of cases, authors judged the intervention effective for certain outcomes but the reviewers disagreed. They judged these interventions to be ineffective or unclear in their effect on these outcomes. The main reasons for disagreement were a high attrition rate (i.e. one-third or more) not adequately dealt with (for example, no information on drop-outs provided) and/or non-significant differences being discussed by the authors as significant results.

Table 6: Agreement/disagreement between authors and reviewers on the conclusions about the effect of interventions on a range of outcomes: sound outcome evaluations (*N* = 15)* only

Authors' versus Reviewers' conclusions	N	%
Agreement		
Effective for some outcomes	11	73
Ineffective for some outcomes	9	60
Disagreement		
Authors: effective for some outcomes; Reviewers: ineffective/unclear	10	66

*Interventions targeted more than one outcome, hence numbers do not add up to 15 studies.

The implication of the analyses presented in Tables 5 and 6 is that purchasers and providers need to be very critical in their use of evidence to inform their decisions on the development and implementation of health promotion services.

Appendix F. Characteristics of the sound and flawed outcome evaluations

Table 7 gives details of the characteristics of all included outcome evaluations with respect to intervention focus, the country where the study was carried out, the intervention types, persons providing the intervention, and the follow-up interval. None of the sound studies was carried out in the UK.

Table 7: Characteristics of the sound (N = 15) and flawed (N = 35) outcome evaluations

	Sound outcome evaluations					Flawed*
	Effective	Effective some group	Ineffective	Unclear	Harmful	Unclear
Country†						
UK	0	0	0	0	0	1
Other Europe	1	0	1	1	0	0
North America	11	0	9	4	1	32
Other	0	0	0	0	0	2
Focus of intervention‡						
Alcohol abuse	4	0	3	1	0	4
Accidents	1	0	1	0	0	7
Cancer	1	0	1	1	0	6
Cardiovascular disease	3	0	2	1	0	10
Healthy eating	6	0	6	3	0	7
Mental health	2	0	1	0	0	8
Physical activity	3	0	2	0	0	9
Smoking	4	0	4	3	0	4
Weight loss	0	0	0	0	0	3
Other	2	0	3	1	1	11
Type of intervention‡						
Advice/counselling	1	0	1	0	0	5
Environmental modification	2	0	2	2	0	7
Exercise	3	0	2	0	0	6
Increased access resources/services	2	0	3	2	0	11
Information/education	10	0	9	4	1	29
Legislation/regulation	1	0	2	2	0	1
Practical skill development	3	0	4	2	0	7
Risk assessment/screening	4	0	4	1	0	21
Social support	2	0	2	1	0	3
Other/unclear	3	0	3	3	0	7

Table 7: Characteristics of the sound (*N* = 15) and flawed (*N* = 35) outcome evaluations (cont'd)

	Sound outcome evaluations					
	Effective	Partially effective	Ineffective	Unclear	Harmful	Flawed* Unclear†
Intervention provider‡						
Community/social worker	1	0	2	0	0	2
Counsellor/psychologist	2	0	2	0	0	0
Health professional	1	0	0	0	0	14
Health promotion practitioner	3	0	3	1	0	6
Peer	4	0	5	1	0	10
Other	3	0	2	3	0	14
Unclear/not relevant	4	0	3	3	1	12
Follow-up interval‡						
< 3 months	7	0	6	3	1	17
3–6 months	2	0	1	0	0	1
7–12 months	3	0	2	2	0	10
> 1 year	4	0	3	2	0	11
None/unclear	0	0	0	0	0	7

*Conclusions cannot be drawn from flawed evaluations, therefore in the reviewers' judgement the impact of the intervention is considered to be unclear.
†Some of the interventions targeted more than one outcome measure, so the numbers do not add up to 50 studies or 100.
‡Some studies included more than one focus of intervention, type of intervention, provider, and/or follow-up interval, as well as a range of outcome measures, hence numbers for these variables do not add up to 50 studies or 100%.

The findings in Table 7 indicate a wide range of interventions in terms of focus, intervention type and intervention provider from which there is no clear pattern emerging with respect to those most successful in changing the targeted outcomes, i.e. behavioural and/or clinical risk factors. Most interventions have been evaluated with respect to short-term effects (i.e. less than 3 months) only; very few have investigated the longer-term maintenance of any changes in targeted outcomes.

There is a clear need to evaluate workplace health promotion interventions further, where feasible, by means of high quality randomised controlled trials.

Appendix G. Description of soundly evaluated interventions

(EPIC number*) Reference	Country	Population	Service provider	Setting	Objectives	Programme content
(3006) Jeffery et al., 1993	USA	40% managerial/professional 40% clerical/sales 20% blue collar workers	Health promotion practitioner	Sites with 400–900 employees in a metropolitan area	To help people stop smoking and lose weight	On-site classes or self-instruction manual combined with incentives through payroll deduction
(3007) Glasgow et al., 1994 (3070) Glasgow et al., 1995 (3069) Terborg, Hibbard, and Glasgow, 1995	USA	50% managerial/professional/technical/sales/clerical; 50% craftsmen/unskilled/service	Community; peer	Sites with 125–750 employees from a range of industry types	To reduce tobacco use, dietary fat intake and cholesterol level	*Take Heart* – 72-page guidebook for site health promotion steering committees to (a) provide encouragement, (b) develop new skills (c) change the worksite or (d) use community resources
(3019) Kronenfeld et al., 1987	USA	23% high school graduates; 29% college/technical education; 22% college graduates; 20% post-bachelor training	Graduate assistants in health education	Employees in public service in South Carolina	To change the behaviour among much of the worksite population, not only those who participated in short courses or special programmes	Comprehensive intervention including programmes for weight control and nutrition, stress management, exercise, smoking cessation, alcohol education and safety education through information/education; physical activity; risk assessment; discussion group sessions; one-to-one communication; printed materials/posters
(3024) Erfurt, Foote and Heirich, 1991a (3060) Erfurt, Foote and Heirich, 1991b (3061) Erfurt, Foote and Heirich, 1992 (3062) Erfurt et al., 1990	USA	85% hourly paid	Health promotion practitioner; counsellor; peer	Manufacturing sites with 1500–3000 employees	To control high blood pressure, obesity and cigarette smoking	Wellness screening; health education; follow-up counselling; menu-approach to wellness activities; health communication networks and support systems
(3030) Parkinson et al., 1989	USA Canada	95% male; approx. 2/3 college graduates	Staff and union members	Operating coke oven plants in the steel industry in the US and Canada	To reduce risk of cancer through increasing awareness and compliance with regulations	Health education sessions: overview of health and safety conditions; occupational cancer surveillance; regulations for personal practice and engineering controls; current state of control at each plant

Appendix G. Description of soundly evaluated interventions (cont'd)

(EPIC number*) Reference	Country	Population	Service provider	Setting	Objectives	Programme content
(3066) Forster et al., 1985 (3055) Forster, Jeffery and Snell, 1988	USA	Faculty; administrative/technical; clerical	Health promotion practitioner	Regular payroll employees of the University of Minnesota	To control weight	Weight loss incentives through payroll deductions; weight loss self-instruction manual and food records for monitoring eating behaviours and calorie intake; weigh-ins and group educational sessions and personal advice
(3067) Jeffery, Forster and Snell, 1985 (3055) Forster, Jeffery and Snell, 1988	USA	22% faculty; 45% administrative/ technical; 33% clerical	Health promotion practitioner	Employees at the School of Public Health/ Medicine at the University of Minnesota	To control weight	Weight loss incentives through payroll deductions; weight loss self-instruction manual and food records for monitoring eating behaviours and calorie intake; weigh-ins and group educational sessions
(3074) Wilbur, Hartwell and Piserchia, 1986	USA	Relatively young; 60% of the men had at least a college education	Health promotion practitioner; peer	Johnson & Johnson plants	To improve health knowledge, nutrition, stress management. To control weight, blood pressure, alcohol consumption, health service use	Live For Life Program: a broad health promotion programme including health screening; lifestyle seminar; lifestyle improvement programmes and environmental modification (exercise facilities, provision of scales, nutritious cafeteria food, car-pooling, smoking policy, health fairs)
(3088) Levin, 1996	USA	Government employees	Environmental modification	Urban worksites in Albuquerque, New Mexico	To increase sales of labelled, low-fat meals and to maintain their increased sales over time	Point-of-purchase intervention programme labeling low-fat meals on the cafeteria menu and organising a raffle
(3089) Brown, 1996	USA	High-pay clerical; medium-pay clerical/ printing company line workers; lower-pay clothing piece workers/ manufacturing and food-processing line workers	Cooperative extension county-based family living agents	Worksites in Pennsylvanian counties	To improve knowledge, attitudes and behaviour related to osteoporosis	Osteoporosis learn-at-home lessons either distributed in an impersonal way, or as part of a motivational meeting

Appendix G. Description of soundly evaluated interventions (cont'd)

(EPIC number*) Reference	Country	Population	Service provider	Setting	Objectives	Programme content
(3093) Brug et al., 1996	The Netherlands	Highly educated compared to the general population	Mailing	Royal Shell laboratory	To reduce fat intake. To increase fruit and vegetable consumption	Dietary intake assessment followed by a letter with computer-generated nutrition advice tailored to the participants' dietary intake, beliefs and awareness levels
(3126) Stoltzfus and Benson, 1994	USA	All employees including site managers and supervisors	Peers; teacher/lecturer; local Employee Assistance Programme contractor and professional	Minnesota Mining and Manufacturing (3M) company	To combat drug and alcohol abuse	A comprehensive alcohol and drug prevention programme including a training component aimed at altering the workplace culture; an educational component for setting personal guidelines; and a skill development peer-helper component
(3135) Sorensen et al., 1996 (3095) Abrams et al., 1994 (3096) Heimendinger et al., 1995	USA	Predominantly blue collar workers including service work, manual labour, machine operation, skill or craft work	Not specified	Worksites representing manufacturing, communications, public service and utilities	To address dietary and smoking behaviour in the context of cancer control through behavioural as well as organisational change	Interventions at individual, community and organisational levels promoting awareness; providing skills for action; and preventing relapse through organisational changes
(3143) Cook, Back and Trudeau, 1996	USA	Predominantly blue collar workers	Counsellor	Medium-sized printing company	To motivate drinkers towards a closer examination of their drinking habits. To reduce alcohol consumption, especially among heavy drinkers. To reduce the amount of heavy drinking among drinkers	Self-efficacy enhancement, improvement of social resistance skills, and bolstering social support
(3148) Sheeshka and Woolcott, 1994	Canada	White collar workers	Not specified	Unionised office and technical employees on a university campus	To promote changes in expectancies, values and intentions related to healthy eating practices and positive health outcomes	Education on the relationship between diet and body weight, cancer, heart disease and osteoporosis; computerised diet analyses, supermarket tours, take-home activities, and group walks

*The number preceding the reference is the unique identifier of the report on the effectiveness database of the EPI-centre

Appendix H. Description of the sound evaluations

(EPIC number) Reference	Design	Nr conditions/ Sample size*	Follow-up interval	Participation rate Attrition	Authors' judgement	Reviewers' judgement
(3006) Jeffery et al., 1993	Randomised controlled trial (RCT)	2 groups; 16 sites each	2 years concurrent with intervention	Participation: 2–10% Attrition: not relevant (before/after surveys)	Effective for smoking Ineffective for weight loss	Unclear for smoking (authors do not take into account differences in smoking policies). Ineffective for weight loss
(3007) Glasgow et al., 1994 (3070) Glasgow et al., 1995 (3069) Terborg, Hibbard and Glasgow, 1995	RCT	2 groups; 13 sites each	2 years concurrent with intervention	Participation 20–40% Attrition: not relevant (before/after surveys)	Ineffective for smoking, fat intake and cholesterol level	Reviewers agreed with authors
(3019) Kronenfeld et al., 1987	Trial	2 groups; 412 employees 313 employees	10 months	Participation 66% Attrition: 30%	Effective for reducing alcohol intake and smoking. Ineffective for dietary habits, exercise behaviour, safety practices, stress and other mental health measures	Reviewers agreed with authors except for the effect on smoking which was judged as unclear due to some baseline differences
(3024) Erfurt, Foote and Heirich, 1991a (3060) Erfurt, Foote and Heirich, 1991b (3061) Erfurt, Foote and Heirich, 1992 (3062) Erfurt et al., 1990	RCT	4 groups; 2448 employees 1374 employees 2089 employees 1893 employees	3 years concurrent with intervention	Participation: 75% to screening alone; 82–88% to screening with other activities Attrition: not relevant (before/after surveys)	Effective for blood pressure control and smoking. Ineffective for weight loss	Reviewers agreed with authors
(3030) Parkinson et al., 1989	RCT	2 groups; 7 sites each	6 months	Participation: not stated Attrition: 10%	Effective for knowledge and self-reported safety practices	Reviewers agreed with authors
(3066) Forster et al., 1985 (3055) Forster, Jeffery and Snell, 1988	RCT	4 groups; G1: 32 employees G2: 29 employees S1: 32 employees S2: 38 employees G = group instruction S = self-instruction	Immediately after intervention	Participation: 4% Attrition: G1: 19%; G2: 21%; S1: 32%; S2: 38%	Weight loss was highest in those using self-instruction and receiving incentives for weight loss; but weight regained within one year	Reviewers agreed with authors

Appendix H. Description of the sound evaluations (cont'd)

(EPIC number) Reference	Design	Nr conditions/ Sample size*	Follow-up interval	Participation rate Attrition	Authors' judgement	Reviewers' judgement
(3067) Jeffery, Forster and Snell, 1985 (3055) Forster, Jeffery and Snell, 1988	RCT	2 groups; 18 employees each	Immediately after intervention	Participation: 6% Attrition: 11% in control group	Effective for weight loss in the short-term, but weight regained within one year	Reviewers agreed with authors
(3074) Wilbur, Hartwell and Piserchia, 1986	Trial	2 groups; 4 sites 3 sites	2 years concurrent with intervention	Participation: 73–79% in screening Attrition: not relevant (before/during/after surveys)	Effective for exercise, tobacco use, stress management, weight control and employee attitudes	Reviewers agreed with authors
(3088) Levin, 1996	Trial	2 groups; 1 site each	Concurrent with intervention: during first 2 weeks; during last 2 weeks; at 6 months (no control group)	Participation: not relevant (worksite as unit of analysis) Attrition: none	Daily sales of targeted low-fat meals increased significantly and the improvement was maintained over 6 months	The maintenance of increased sales at 6 months follow-up was unclear, because no data were collected in the control site
(3089) Brown, 1996	Trial	3 groups; G: 114 employees I: 114 employees C: 125 employees	2 weeks 4 months	Participation: no data on eligible population Attrition: G: 30%; I: 24%; C: 36%	Effective for knowledge, with knowledge increase significantly higher in the group-delivery condition compared to the impersonal delivery condition. Effective for reported behaviour 2 weeks after the intervention; maintained at 4 months follow-up in the group-delivery condition only; calcium intake was not significantly different between group-delivery and impersonal delivery conditions. Ineffective for attitudes	Reviewers agreed with authors

Appendix H. Description of the sound evaluations (cont'd)

(EPIC number) Reference	Design	Nr conditions/ Sample size*	Follow-up interval	Participation rate Attrition	Authors' judgement	Reviewers' judgement
(3093) Brug et al., 1996	RCT	2 groups; 507 employees, approx. half in each group	3 weeks	Participation: 74% Attrition: 32% overall; no difference between groups	Effective for attitudes towards vegetable/fruit consumption. Ineffective for attitudes to fat intake. Effective for intentions to change diet. Ineffective for beliefs/ self-efficacy. Effective for fat/vegetable intake. Ineffective for fruit consumption	Reviewers agreed with authors except for the attitude changes which reviewers judged as unclear
(3126) Stoltzfus and Benson, 1994	Trial	2 groups; I: 445 employees C: 214 employees	3 months 16 months (no control group)	Participation: not voluntary Attrition: I: 7% at 3 months; 9% at 16 months; no attrition in control group	Effective for alcohol use (frequency and amount); drinking and driving; riding with a driver under influence; impact of alcohol on work. Effective for 10-item at risk-index. Ineffective for marijuana and smokeless tobacco use (probably due to very low baseline levels)	The maintenance of behaviour changes and improvement in attitudes and self-efficacy at 16 months follow-up were unclear, due to the lack of a control group
(3135) Sorensen et al., 1996 (3095) Abrams et al., 1994 (3096) Heimendinger et al., 1995	RCT	2 groups; 54 sites each	1 year	Participation: 72% Attrition: not stated	Effective for fat/fruit/ vegetable consumption. Ineffective for smoking. Ineffective for fat/fruit/ vegetable consumption. Ineffective for smoking	
(3143) Cook, Back and Trudeau, 1996	Trial	3 groups; I: 50 employees on-site C: 60 employees off-site C: 50 employees	Immediately after intervention	Participation: 26% Attrition: I: 24%; on-site C: 57% off-site C: 12%	Ineffective for health beliefs; moving through stages of change; self-efficacy for drinking reduction; experiencing problems at work due to alcohol; average number of drinks on drinking days decrease alcohol use; number of drinking days and heavy drinking,	Reviewers agreed with authors
(3148) Sheeshka and Woolcott, 1994	Trial	2 groups: I: 26 employees C: 25 employees	Immediately after intervention	Participation: 61% Attrition: I: 18.5%; C: 8%	Effective for self-efficacy; and partially effective for attitudes. Ineffective for intentions to adopt healthy eating	Reviewers agreed with authors

* I = Intervention group; C = Control/comparison group

Appendix I. Included studies

<<EPIC number>>
(unique identifier of the report on EPIC, the EPI-Centre effectiveness database)

** sound evaluations
* flawed evaluations

Abrams, D B, Boutwell, W B, Grizzle J, Heimendinger, J, Sorensen, G and Varnes, J (1994). Cancer control at the workplace: the Working Well trial. *Preventive Medicine* **23**:15–27.
** <<EPIC 3095 linked to 3096 & 3135>>

Allegrante, J P and Michela, J L (1990). Impact of school-workplace health promotion program on morale of inner-city school teachers. *Journal of School Health* **60**(1):25–8.
* <<EPIC 3032 >>

Baier, C A, Grodzin, C J, Port, J D, Leksas, L and Tancredi, D J (1992). Coronary risk factor behavior change in hospital personnel following a screening program. *American Journal of Preventive Medicine* **8**(2):115–22.
* <<EPIC 3028 >>

Blair, S N, Piserchia, P V, Wilbur, C S and Crowder, J H (1986). A public health intervention model for work-site health promotion: impact on exercise and physical fitness in a health promotion plan after 24 months. *Journal of the American Medical Association* **255**:921–6.
* <<EPIC 3076 linked to 3054, 3033, 3074 & 3075 >>

Blake, S M, Casperson, C J, Finnegan, J, Crow, R A, Mittlemark, M B and Ringhofer, K R (1996). The Shape Up Challenge: a community-based worksite exercise competition. *American Journal of Health Promotion* **11**(1):23–34.
* <<EPIC 3105 >>

Bly, J L, Jones, R C and Richardson, J E (1986). Impact of worksite health promotion on health care costs and utilization: evaluation of Johnson and Johnson's Live for Life program. *Journal of the American Medical Association* **256**:3235–40.
* <<EPIC 3003 >>

Brown, J L (1996). Effect of delivery method on impact of learn-at-home lessons at worksites. *Journal of Nutrition Education* **28**(3):140–8.
** <<EPIC 3089 >>

Brownell, K D, Cohen, R Y, Stunkard, A J, Felix, M R J and Cooley, N B (1984). Weight loss competitions at the work site: impact on weight, morale, and cost-effectiveness. *American Journal of Public Health* **74**(11):1283–5.
* <<EPIC 3025 >>

Brug, J, Steenhuis, I, Van Assema, P and De Vries, H (1996). The impact of a computer-tailored nutrition intervention. *Preventive Medicine* **25**:236–42.
** <<EPIC 3093 >>

Calladine, Mary L (1996). Nursing process for health promotion using King's theory. *Journal of Community Health Nursing* **13**(1):51–7.
* <<EPIC 3116 >>

Chavalinitikul, N, Nopteepkangwan, N and Kanjanopas, F (1995). Improvement of lifting heavy objects at work. *Journal of Human Ergology* **24**:55–8.
* <<EPIC 3101 >>

Chilcote, W A, Barry, M, Paushter, D M, Desberg, A, Churchill, E and Jeric, R (1994). Patient initiated breast cancer screening: results of a comprehensive community and workplace sponsored program. *Breast Disease* **7**:151–6.
* <<EPIC 3130 >>

Cook, R F, Back, A S and Trudeau, J (1996). Preventing alcohol use problems among blue-collar workers: a field test of the Working People program. *Substance Use and Misuse* **31**(3):255–75.
★★ <<EPIC 3143 >>

Cooper, M D, Phillips, R A, Sutherland, V J and Makin, P J (1994). Reducing accidents using goal setting and feedback: a field study. *Journal of Occupational and Organizational Psychology* **67**(3):219–40.
★ <<EPIC 3140 >>

Daltroy, L H, Iversen, M D, Larson, M G, Ryan, J, Zwerling, C, Fossel, A H and Liang, M H (1993). Teaching and social support: effects on knowledge, attitudes and behaviors to prevent low back injuries in industry. *Health Education Quarterly* **20**(1):43–62.
★ <<EPIC 3023 >>

Davis, E and Johnson, M (1994). Lower back disability in the campus setting: a longitudinal study. *CUPA Journal* **45**(3):13–19.
★ <<EPIC 3137 >>

Erfurt, J C, Foote, A, Heirich, M A and Gregg, W (1990). Improving participation in worksite wellness programs: company health education classes, a menu approach, and follow-up counseling. *American Journal of Health Promotion* **4**:270–8.
★★ <<EPIC 3062 linked to 3024, 3060 & 3061 >>

Erfurt, J C, Foote, A and Heirich, M (1991a). Worksite wellness programs: incremental comparison of screening and referral alone, health education, follow-up counseling, and plant organisation. *American Journal of Health Promotion* **5**:438–48.
★★ <<EPIC 3024 linked to 3060, 3061 & 3062 >>

Erfurt, J C, Foote, A and Heirich, M A (1991b). The cost-effectiveness of worksite wellness programs for hypertension control, weight loss, and smoking cessation. *Journal of Occupational Medicine* **33**(9):962–70.
★★ <<EPIC 3060 linked to 3024, 3061 & 3062 >>

Erfurt, J C, Foote, A and Heirich, M A (1992). The cost-effectiveness of worksite wellness programs for hypertension control, weight loss, smoking cessation and exercise. *Personnel Psychology* **45**:5–27.
★★ <<EPIC 3061 linked to 3024, 3060 & 3062 >>

Felner, R D, Brand, S, Mulhall, K E, Counter, B, Millman, J B and Fried, J (1994). The parenting partnership: the evaluation of a human service/corporate workplace collaboration for the prevention of substance abuse and mental health problems, and the promotion of family and work adjustment. *Journal of Primary Prevention* **15**(2):123–46.
★ <<EPIC 3125 >>

Fielding, J E, Knight, K, Mason, T, Klesges, R C and Pelletier, K R (1994). Evaluation of the IMPACT blood pressure program. *Journal of Occupational and Environmental Medicine* **36**(7):743–6.
★ <<EPIC 3086 >>

Fielding, J E, Mason, T, Knight, K, Klesges, R and Pelletier, K R (1995). A randomized trial of the IMPACT worksite cholesterol reduction program. *American Journal of Preventive Medicine* **11**(2):120–3.
★ <<EPIC 3100 >>

Fisher, S P and Fisher, M M (1995). Development, implementation, and evaluation of a health promotion program in a college setting. *Journal of American College Health* **44**:81–3.
★ <<EPIC 3108 >>

Forster, J L, Jeffery, R W, Sullivan, S and Snell, M K (1985). A work-site weight control program using financial incentives collected through payroll deduction. *Journal of Occupational Medicine* **27**(11):804–8.
★★ <<EPIC 3066 linked to 3055 >>

Forster, J L, Jeffery, R W and Snell, M K (1988). One-year follow-up study to a worksite weight control program. *Preventive Medicine* **17**:129–33.
★★ <<EPIC 3055 linked to 3066 & 3067 >>

Frampton, S B, Brochu, S and Murray, J (1996). Creative strategies for promotion of worksite health services: The Employee Ambassador Program. *American Journal of Health Promotion* **11**(1):10–11.
★ <<EPIC 3103 >>

Garofalo, K (1994). Worksite wellness – rewarding healthy behaviors: successful program. *AAOHN Journal* **42**(5):236–40.
★ <<EPIC 3120 >>

Glasgow, R E, Terborg, J R, Hollis, J F *et al.* (1994). Modifying dietary and tobacco use patterns in the worksite: the Take Heart project. *Health Education Quarterly* **21**(1):69–82.
★★ <<EPIC 3007 linked to 3069 & 3070 >>

Glasgow, R E, Terborg, J R, Hollis, J F, Severson, H H and Boles, S M (1995). Take Heart: results from the initial phase of work-site Wellness Program. *American Journal of Public Health* **85**(2):209–16.
★★ <<EPIC 3070 linked to 3007 & 3069 >>

Greenwood, M and Henritze, J (1996). Coorscreen: a low-cost, on-site mammography screening program. *American Journal of Health Promotion* **10**(5):364–71.
★ <<EPIC 3147 >>

Guldan, G S, Zhang, Y, Huang, Y, Yang, X and Zeng, G (1992). Effectiveness of a worksite education activity in a factory in China. *Asia Pacific Journal of Public Health* **6**(2):8–14.
★ <<EPIC 3034 >>

Hartman, T J, McCarthy, P R and Himes, J H (1993). Use of eating pattern messages to evaluate eating behaviors in a worksite cholesterol education program. *American Dietetic Association Journal* **93**(10):1119–23.
★ <<EPIC 3038 linked to 3082 >>

Hartman, T J, Himes, J H, McCarthy, P R and Kushi, L H (1995). Effects of a low-fat, worksite intervention on blood lipids and lipoproteins. *Journal of Occupational and Environmental Medicine* **37**(6):690–6.
★ <<EPIC 3082 linked to 3038 >>

Heaney, C A (1991). Enhancing social support at the workplace assessing the effects of the Caregiver Support Program. *Health Education Quarterly* **18**(4):477–94.
★ <<EPIC 3029 >>

Hebert, J R, Stoddard, A M, Harris, D R *et al.* (1993). Measuring the effect of a worksite-based nutrition intervention on food consumption. *Association of Educational Psychologists* **3**(6):629–35.
★ <<EPIC 3064 linked to 3052, 3063 & 3065 >>

Heimendinger, J, Feng, Z, Emmons, K *et al.* (1995). The Working Well Trial: baseline dietary and smoking behaviors of employees and related worksite characteristics. *Preventive Medicine* **24**:180–93.
★★ <<EPIC 3096 linked to 3095 & 3135 >>

Holbrook, M I, White, M H and Hutt, M J (1994). Increasing awareness of sleep hygiene in rotating shift workers: arming law-enforcement officers against impaired performance. *Perception Motor Skills* **79**(1, pt 2):520–2.
★ <<EPIC 3145 >>

Holzbach, R L, Piserchia, P V, McFadden, D W *et al.* (1990) Effect of a comprehensive health promotion program on employee attitudes. *Journal of Occupational Medicine* **32**(10):973–8.
★ <<3054 linked to 3033, 3074, 3075 & 3076 >>

Hornsby, P P, Reeve, R H, Gwaltney, J M Jr, Parsons, B D and Morse, R M (1997). The University of Virginia health promotion and disease prevention program. *American Journal of Preventive Medicine* **13**(1):36–44.
★ <<EPIC 3128>>

Huddy, D C, Herbert, J L, Hyner, G C and Johnson, R L (1995). Facilitating changes in exercise behavior: effect of structured statements of intention on perceived barriers to action. *Psychological Reports* **76**(3):867–75.
★ <<EPIC 3146>>

Jeffery, R W, Forster, J L and Snell, M K (1985). Promoting weight control at the worksite: a pilot program of self-motivation using payroll based incentives. *Preventive Medicine* **14**:187–94.
★★ <<EPIC 3067 linked to 3055>>

Jeffery, R W, Forster, J L and Schmid, T L (1989). Worksite health promotion: feasibility testing of repeated weight control and smoking cessation classes. *American Journal of Health Promotion* **3**(4):11–16.
★ <<EPIC 3072>>

Jeffery, R W, Forster, J L, French, S A *et al.* (1993). The Healthy Worker Project: a worksite intervention for weight control and smoking cessation. *American Journal of Public Health* **83**(3):395–401.
★★ <<EPIC 3006>>

Jones, R C, Bly, J L and Richardson, J E (1990). A study of a work site health promotion program and absenteeism. *Journal of Occupational Medicine* **32**(2):95–9.
★ <<EPIC 3014>>

Kishchuk, N, Peters, C, Towers, A M, Sylvestre, M and Bourgault, R L (1994). Formative and effectiveness evaluation of a worksite program promoting healthy alcohol consumption. *American Journal of Health Promotion* **8**(5):353–62.
★ <<EPIC 3091 linked to 3149>>

Kronenfeld, J J, Jackson, K, Blair, S N *et al.* (1987). Evaluating health promotion: a longitudinal quasi-experimental design. *Health Education Quarterly* **14**(2):123–39.
★★ <<EPIC 3019>>

Levin, S (1996). Pilot study of a cafeteria program relying primarily on symbols to promote healthy choices. *Journal of Nutrition Education* **28**(5):282–5.
★★ <<EPIC 3088>>

McQuiston, T H, Coleman, P, Wallerstein, N B, Marcus, A C, Morawetz, J S and Ortlieb, D W (1994). Hazardous waste worker education. *Journal of Occupational Medicine* **36**(12):1310–23.
★ <<EPIC 3133>>

Nelson, D J, Sennett, L and Lefebre, R C (1987). A campaign strategy for weight loss at worksites. *Health Education Research* **2**(1):27–31.
★ <<EPIC 3037>>

Parkinson, D K, Bromet, E J, Dew, M A, Dunn, L O, Barkman, M and Wright, M (1989). Effectiveness of the united steel workers of America coke oven intervention program. *Journal of Occupational Medicine* **31**(5):464–72.
★★ <<EPIC 3030>>

Saari, J, Bedard, S, Dufort, V, Hryniewiecki, J and Theriault, G (1994). Successful training strategies to implement a workplace hazardous materials information system. *Journal of Occupational Medicine* **36**(5):569–74.
★ <<EPIC 3094>>

Sheeshka, J D and Woolcott, D M (1994). An evaluation of a theory-based demonstration worksite nutrition promotion program. *American Journal of Health Promotion* **8**(4):263–4, 253.
★★ <<EPIC 3148>>

Shipley, R H, Orleans, C T, Wilbur, C S, Piserchia, P V and McFadden, D W (1988). Effect of the Johnson and Johnson Live for Life program on employee smoking. *Preventive Medicine* **17**:25–34.
★ <<EPIC 3033 linked to 3054, 3074, 3075 & 3076>>

Sorensen, G, Hunt, M K, Morris, D H *et al.* (1990). Promoting healthy eating patterns in the worksite: the Treatwell intervention model. *Health Education Research* **5**(4):505–15.
★ <<EPIC 3065 linked to 3052, 3063 & 3064>>

Sorensen, G, Hsieh, J, Hunt, M K, Morris, D H and Fitzgerald, G (1992a). Employee advisory boards as a vehicle for organizing worksite health promotion programs. *American Journal of Health Promotion* **6**(6):443–50.
★ <<EPIC 3063 linked to 3052, 3064 & 3065>>

Sorensen, G, Morris D M, Hunt, M *et al.* (1992b). Work-site nutrition intervention and employees' dietary habits: the Treatwell program. *American Journal of Public Health* **82**(6):877–80.
★ <<EPIC 3052 linked to 3063, 3064 & 3065>>

Sorensen, G, Thompson, B, Glanz, K *et al.* (1996). Work site-based cancer prevention: primary results from the Working Well Trial. *American Journal of Public Health* **86**(7):939–47.
★★ <<EPIC 3135 linked to 3095 & 3096>>

Stevens, M M, Paine-Andrews, A and Francisco, V T (1996). Improving employee health and wellness: a pilot study of the employee-driven Perfect Health Program. *American Journal of Health Promotion* **11**(1):12–14.
★ <<EPIC 3104>>

Stoffelmayr, B E, Mavis, B E, Stachnik, T, Robison, J, Rogers, M, Vanhuss, W and Carlson, J (1992). A program model to enhance adherence in work-site-based fitness programs. *Journal of Occupational Medicine* February:156–61.
★ <<EPIC 3036>>

Stoltzfus, J A and Benson, P L (1994). The 3M alcohol and other drug prevention program: description and evaluation. *Journal of Primary Prevention* **15**(2):147–59.
★★ <<EPIC 3126>>

Terborg, J R, Hibbard, J and Glasgow, R E (1995). Behavior change at the worksite: Does social support make a difference? *American Journal of Public Health* **10**(2):125–31.
★★ <<EPIC 3069 linked to 3007 & 3070>>

Towers, A M, Kishchuk, N, Sylvestre, M, Peters, C and Bourgault, C (1994). A qualitative investigation of organizational issues in an alcohol awareness program for blue-collar workers. *American Journal of Health Promotion* **9**(1):56–63.
★ <<EPIC 3149 linked to 3091>>

Wilbur, C S (1983). Live for Life: the Johnson & Johnson program. *Preventive Medicine* **12**:672–81.
★ <<EPIC 3075 linked to 3033, 3054, 3074 & 3076>>

Wilbur, C S, Hartwell, T D, Piserchia, P V (1986). The Johnson and Johnson Live for Life program: its organization and evaluation plan. In: Cataldo, M F and Coates, T J (eds). *Health and Industry*. New York: John Wiley & Sons, p. 338–350.
★★ <<EPIC 3074 linked to 3033, 3054, 3075 & 3076>>

Wong, Y T, Bauman, K E and Koch, G G (1996). Increasing low income employee participation in a worksite health promotion program: a comparison of three common strategies. *Health Education Research* **11**(1):71–6.
★ <<EPIC 3113>>

Zimmerman, R S, Safer, M A, Leventhal, H and Baumann, L J (1986). The effects of health information in a worksite hypertension screening program. *Health Education Quarterly* **13**(3):261–80.
★ <<EPIC 3057>>

Appendix J. Excluded studies

<<EPIC number>>

(unique identifier of the report on EPIC, the EPI-Centre effectiveness database)

Abrams, D B and Follick, M J (1983). Behavioral weight-loss intervention at the worksite: feasibility and maintenance. *Journal of Consulting and Clinical Psychology* **51**(2):226–33.
<<EPIC 3039>>

Aldana, S G, Jacobson, B H, Harris, C J and Kelley, P L (1993). Mobile work-site health promotion programs can reduce selected employee health risks. *Journal of Occupational Medicine* **35**(9):922–8.
<<EPIC 3026>>

Aldana, S G, Jacobson, B H, Kelley, P L and Quirk, M (1994). The effectiveness of a mobile worksite health promotion program in lowering employee health risk. *American Journal of Health Promotion* 8(4):254–6.
<<EPIC 3090>>

Amos, A, White, D A and Elton, R (1995). Is a telephone helpline of value to the workplace smoker? *Occupational Medicine* **45**(5):234–8.
<<EPIC 3158>>

Anderson, R C and Anderson, K E (1994). Positive changes and worksite health education. *Psychological Reports* **74**(2):607–10.
<<EPIC 3127>>

Arnetz, B B (1996). Techno-Stress: a prospective psychophysiological study of the impact of a controlled stress-reduction program in advanced telecommunications systems design work. *Journal of Occupational and Environmental Medicine* **38**(1):53–65.
<<EPIC 3119>>

Barratt, A, Reznik, R, Irwig, L *et al.* (1994). Work-site cholesterol screening and dietary intervention: the Staff Healthy Heart Project. *American Journal of Public Health* **84**(5):779–82.
<<EPIC 3098>>

Bertera, R, Oehl, L and Telepchak, J (1990). Self-help versus group approaches to smoking cessation in the workplace: eighteen-month follow-up and cost analysis. *American Journal of Health Promotion* **4**:187–92.
<<EPIC 3040>>

Borland, R, Chapman, S, Owen, N and Hill, D (1990). Effects of workplace smoking bans on cigarette consumption. *American Journal of Public Health* **80**(2):178–80.
<<EPIC 3020>>

Borland, R and Owen, N (1995). Need to smoke in the context of workplace smoking bans. *Preventive Medicine* **24**:56–60.
<<EPIC 3167>>

Boudreau, F, Godin, G, Pineau, R and Bradet, R (1995). Health risk appraisal in an occupational setting and its impact on exercise behavior. *Journal of Occupational and Environmental Medicine* **37**(9):1145–50.
<<EPIC 3080>>

Brenner, H, Born, J, Novak, P and Waner, V (1997). Smoking behavior and attitude toward smoking regulations and passive smoking in the workplace. *Preventive Medicine* **26**:138–43.
<<EPIC 3150>>

Brenner H and Fleischle B (1994). Smoking regulations at the workplace and smoking behavior: a study from southern Germany. *Preventive Medicine* **23**:230–4.
<<EPIC 3164>>

Brigham, J, Gross, J, Stitzer, M L and Felch, L J (1994). Effects of a restricted work-site smoking policy on employees who smoke. *American Journal of Public Health* **84**(5):773–8.
<<EPIC 3160>>

Briley, M E, Montgomery, D H and Blewett, J (1992). Worksite nutrition education can lower total cholesterol levels and promote weight loss among police department employees. *American Dietetic Association Journal* **92**(11):1382–4.
<<EPIC 3044 linked to 3115>>

Byers, T, Mullis, R, Anderson, J *et al.* (1995). The costs and effects of a nutritional education program following work-site cholesterol screening. *American Journal of Public Health* **85**(5):650–5.
<<EPIC 3106>>

Cohen, R and Mrtek, M B (1994). The impact of two corporate lactation programs on the incidence and duration of breast-feeding by employed mothers. *American Journal of Health Promotion* **8**(6):436–41.
<<EPIC 3138>>

Cohen, R, Mrtek, M B and Mrtek, R G (1995). Comparison of maternal absenteeism and infant illness rates among breast-feeding and formula-feeding women in two corporations. *American Journal of Health Promotion* **10**(2):148–53.
<<EPIC 3156>>

Connell, C M, Sharpe, P A and Gallant, M P (1995). Effect of health risk appraisal on health outcomes in a university worksite health promotion trial. *Health Education Research* **10**(2):199–209.
<<EPIC 3118>>

Conrad, K M, Campbell, R T, Edington, D W, Faust, H S and Vilnius, D (1996). The worksite environment as a cue to smoking reduction. *Research in Nursing & Health* **19**(1):21–31.
<<EPIC 3136>>

Daley, A J and Parfitt, G (1996). Good health – is it worth it? Mood states, physical wellbeing, job satisfaction and absenteeism in members and non-members of a British corporate health and fitness club. *Journal of Occupational and Organizational Psychology* **69**(2):121–34.
<<EPIC 3144>>

Daughton, D M, Patil, K D and Rennard, S I (1990). Smoking cessation in the workplace: evaluation of relapse factors. *Preventive Medicine* **19**(2):227–30.
<<EPIC 3049>>

Drazen, M, Nevid, J S, Pace, N and O'Brien, R M (1982). Worksite based behavioral treatment of mild hypertension. *Journal of Occupational Medicine* **24**(7):511–14.
<<EPIC 3043>>

Ellis, E, Koblin, W, Irvine, M J, Legare, J and Logan, A G (1994). Small, blue collar work site hypertension screening: a cost-effectiveness study. *Journal of Occupational and Environmental Medicine* **36**(3):346–55.
<<EPIC 3087>>

Elton, P J, Ryman, A, Hammer, M and Page, F (1994). Randomised controlled trial in northern England of the effect of a person knowing their own serum cholesterol concentration. *Journal of Epidemiology and Community Health* **48**(1):22–5.
<<EPIC 3047>>

Emont, S L and Cummings, K M (1992). Using a low-cost, prize-drawing incentive to improve recruitment rate at a work-site smoking cessation clinic. *Journal of Occupational Medicine* **34**(8):771–5.
<<EPIC 3016>>

Emont, S L, Zahniser, C, Marcus, S E *et al.* (1995). Evaluation of the 1990 Centers for Disease Control and Prevention Smoke Free Policy. *American Journal of Health Promotion* **9**(6):456–461.
<<EPIC 3114>>

Fisher, E B, Bishop, D B, Levitt-Gilmour, T, Cappello, M T, Ashenberg, Z S and Newman, E (1994). Social support in worksite smoking cessation: qualitative analysis of the EASE project. *American Journal of Health Promotion* **9**(1):39–46.
<<EPIC 3159>>

Fitzgerald, S T, Gibbens, S and Agnew, J (1991). Evaluation of referral completion after a workplace cholesterol screening program. *American Journal of Preventive Medicine* **7**(6):335–40.
<<EPIC 3021>>

Friesen, C A and Hoerr, SL (1990). Nutrition education strategies for work-site wellness: evaluation of a graduate course targeted to work-site wellness majors. *American Dietetic Association Journal* **90**(6):854–6.
<<EPIC 3017>>

Gemson, D H and Sloan, R P (1995). Efficacy of computerized health risk appraisal as part of a periodic health examination at the worksite. *American Journal of Health Promotion* **9**(6):462–6.
<<EPIC 3139>>

Gettman, L (1986). Cost/benefit anlysis of a corporate fitness program. *Fitness in Business* **1**:11–17.
<<EPIC 3058>>

Girgis, A, Sanson-Fisher, R W and Watson, A (1994). A workplace intervention for increasing outdoor workers' use of solar protection. *American Journal of Public Health* **84**(1):77–81.
<<EPIC 3035>>

Glasgow, R E, Klesges, R C, Godding, P R, Vasey, M W and O'Neil, H K (1984). Evaluation of a work-site controlled smoking program. *Journal of Consulting and Clinical Psychology* **52**(1):137–8.
<<EPIC 3027>>

Glasgow, R E, Hollis, J F, Ary, D V and Lando, H A (1990). Employee and organizational factors associated with participation in an incentive-based worksite smoking cessation program. *Journal of Behavioral Medicine* **13**:403–18.
<<EPIC 3059>>

Glasgow, R E, Sorensen, G, Giffen, C, Shipley, R H, Corbett, K and Lynn, W (1996). Promoting worksite smoking control policies and actions: the Community Intervention Trial for smoking cessation (COMMIT) experience. *Preventive Medicine* **25**:186–94.
<<EPIC 3162>>

Goetzel, R, Sepulveda, M, Knight, K *et al.* (1994). Association of IBM's 'A Plan for Life' health promotion program with changes in employees' health risk status. *Journal of Occupational and Environmental Medicine* **36**(9):1005–9.
<<EPIC 3083>>

Goetzel, R Z, Kahr, T Y, Aldana, S G and Kenny, G M (1996). An evaluation of Duke University's Live for Life Health Promotion Program and its impact on employee health. *American Journal of Health Promotion* **10**(5):340–1.
<<EPIC 3085>>

Gomel, M, Oldenburg, B, Simpson, J M and Owen, N (1993). Work-site cardiovascular risk reduction: a randomised trial of health risk assessment, education, counselling and incentives. *American Journal of Public Health* **83**(9):1231–8.
<<EPIC 3001 linked to 3002>>

Hammond, S K, Sorensen, G, Youngstrom, R and Ockene, J K (1995). Occupational exposure to environmental tobacco smoke. *Journal of the American Medical Association* **274**(12):956–60.
<<EPIC 3151>>

Haus, G, Hoerr, S L, Mavis, B and Robison, J (1994). Key modifiable factors in weight maintenance: fat intake, exercise, and weight cycling. *American Dietetic Association Journal* **49**(4):409–13.
<<EPIC 3132>>

Heaney, C A and Inglish, P (1995). Are employees who are at risk for cardiovascular disease joining worksite fitness centers? *Journal of Occupational and Environmental Medicine* **37**(6):718–24.
<<EPIC 3081>>

Hudzinski, L G and Sirois, A (1994). Changes in smoking behavior and body weight after implementation of a no-smoking policy in the workplace. *Southern Medical Journal* **87**(3):322–7.
<<EPIC 3129>>

Jason, L A, Gruder, C L, Buckenberger, L *et al.* (1987). A 12-month follow-up of a worksite smoking cessation intervention. *Health Education Research* **2**(3):185–94.
<<EPIC 3022>>

Jeffery, R W, Pheley, A M, Forster, J L, Kramer, F M and Snell, M K (1988). Payroll contracting for smoking cessation; a worksite pilot study. *American Journal of Preventive Medicine* **4**(2):83–4.
<<EPIC 3048>>

Jeffery, R W, Forster, J L and Schmid, T L (1989). Worksite health promotion: feasibility testing of repeated weight control and smoking cessation classes. *American Journal of Health Promotion* **3**:11–16.
<<EPIC 3072>>

Klesges, R, Vasey, M and Glasgow, R (1986). A worksite smoking modification competition: potential for public health impact. *American Journal of Public Health* **76**:198–200.
<<EPIC 3051>>

Kline, M L (1994). Effects of a worksite coping skills intervention on the stress, social support and health outcomes of working mothers. *Journal of Primary Prevention* **15**(2):105–21.
<<EPIC 3111>>

Knight, K K, Goetzel, R Z, Fielding, J E *et al.* (1994). An evaluation of Duke University's Live for Life health promotion program on changes in worker absenteeism. *Journal of Occupational and Environmental Medicine* **36**(5):533–6.
<<EPIC 3084>>

Kornitzer, M, Boutsen, M, Thijs, J and Gustavsson, G (1995). Combined use of nicotine patch and gum in smoking cessation: a placebo-controlled clinical trial. *Preventive Medicine* **24**:41–7.
<<EPIC 3165>>

Longo, D, Brownson, R and Kruse, R (1995). Smoking bans in US hospitals: results of a national survey. *Journal of the American Medical Association* **274**(6):488–91.
<<EPIC 3152>>

Longo, D R, Brownson, R C, Johnson, J C *et al.* (1996). Hospital smoking bans and employee smoking behavior: results of a national survey. *Journal of the American Medical Association* **275**(16):1252–7.
<<EPIC 3123>>

Maheu, M M, Gevirtz, R N, Sallis, J F and Schneider, N (1989). Competition/cooperation in worksite smoking cessation using nicotine gum. *Preventive Medicine* **18**:867–76.
<<EPIC 3046>>

Malott, J M, Glasgow, R E, O'Neill, H K and Klesges, R C (1984). Co-worker social support in a worksite smoking control program. *Journal of Applied Behavior Analysis* **17**(4):485–95.
<<EPIC 3041>>

Mankani, S K, Garabrant, D H and Homa, D M (1996). Effectiveness of nicotine patches in a workplace smoking cessation program. *Journal of Occupational and Environmental Medicine* **38**(2):184–9.
<<EPIC 3166>>

Martin, J P (1990). Male cancer awareness: impact of an employee education program. *Oncology Nursing Forum* **17**(1):59–64.
<<EPIC 3045>>

McCann, K B and Sulzer-Azaroff, B (1996). Cumulative trauma disorders: behavioral injury prevention at work. *Journal of Applied Behavioral Science* **32**(3):277–91.
<<EPIC 3141>>

Melhorn, J M (1996). A prospective study for upper-extremity cumulative trauma disorders of workers in aircraft manufacturing. *Journal of Occupational and Environmental Medicine* **38**(12):1264.
<<EPIC 3121>>

Montgomery, D H and Briley, M E (1995). Long-term dietary intake changes in police department employees who participated in a worksite nutrition education program. *Clinical Nutrition* **10**(4):78–84.
<<EPIC 3115 linked to 3044>>

Murakami, M, Katsura, T, Sasaki Y *et al.* (1996) Evaluation and promotion of mental health for industrial hygiene. *Japanese Journal of Psychosomatic Medicine* **36**:161–7.
<<EPIC 3142>>

Murphy, L R (1983). A comparison of relaxation methods for reducing stress in nursing personnel. *Human Factors* **25**(4):431–40.
<<EPIC 3031>>

Oldenburg, B, Owen, N, Parle, M and Gomel, M (1995). An economic evaluation of four work site based cardiovascular risk factor interventions. *Health Education Quarterly* **22**(1):9–19.
<<EPIC 3002 linked to 3001>>

Olson, G M, Pellien, A, Maroney, G *et al.* (1991). An analysis of the effectiveness of a low back health education program in an employee population. *Journal of Health Education* **22**(3):160–5.
<<EPIC 3008>>

Ostwald, S K (1989). Changing employees' dietary and exercise practices: an experimental study in a small company. *Journal of Occupational Medicine* **31**(2):90–7.
<<EPIC 3012>>

Pederson, L L, Bull, S B and Ashley, M J (1996). Smoking in the workplace: do smoking patterns and attitudes reflect the legislative environment? *Tobacco Control* **5**(1):39–45.
<<EPIC 3154>>

Perovich, S and Sandoval, W (1995). Outcomes of a worksite cholesterol education program over a 5-year period. *American Dietetic Association Journal* **95**(5):589–90.
<<EPIC 3112>>

Peters, R K, Benson, H and Porter, D (1977). Daily relaxation response breaks in a working population: I. Effects on self-reported measures of health, performance, and well-being. *American Journal of Public Health* **67**(10):946–53.
<<EPIC 3071 linked to 3000>>

Peters, R K, Benson, H and Peters, J M (1977). Daily relaxation response breaks in a working population: II. Effects on blood pressure. *American Journal of Public Health* **67**(10):954–9.
<<EPIC 3000 linked to 3071>>

Pronk, S J, Pronk, N P, Sisco, A, Ingalls, D S and Ochoa, C (1995). Impact of daily 10-minute strength and flexibility program in a manufacturing plant (pilot study). *American Journal of Health Promotion* **9**(3):175–8.
<<EPIC 3092/3134>>

Pruitt, R H (1992). Effectiveness and cost efficiency of interventions in health promotion. *Journal of Advanced Nursing* **17**(8):926–32.
<<EPIC 3015>>

Pucci, L G and Haglund, B (1994). 'Naturally Smoke free': a support program for facilitating worksite smoking control policy implementation in Sweden. *Health Promotion International* **9**(3):177–87.
<<EPIC 3124>>

Rigotti, N A, Bourne, D, Rosen, A, Locke, J A and Schelling, T C (1992). Workplace compliance with a no-smoking law: a randomized community intervention trial. *American Journal of Public Health* **82**(2):227–35.
<<EPIC 3004>>

Rigotti, N A, Stoto, M A and Schelling, T C (1994). Do businesses comply with a no-smoking law? Assessing the self-enforcement approach. *Preventive Medicine* **23**:223–9.
<<EPIC 3163>>

Ryan, J, Zwerling, C and Jones, M (1996). Cigarette smoking at hire as a predictor of employment outcome. *Journal of Occupational and Environmental Medicine* **38**(9):928–33.
<<EPIC 3122>>

Salina, D, Jason, L A, Hedeker, D *et al.* (1994). A follow-up of a media-based, worksite smoking cessation program. *American Journal of Community Psychology* **22**(2):257–71.
<<EPIC 3155>>

Scott, R, Denier, C A, Prue, D M and King, A C (1986). Worksite smoking intervention with nursing professionals: long-term outcome and relapse assessment. *Journal of Consulting and Clinical Psychology* **54**(6):809–13.
<<EPIC 3056>>

Sherman, J B, Clark, L and McEwen, M M (1989). Evaluation of a worksite wellness program: impact on exercise, weight, smoking and stress. *Public Health Nursing* **6**(3):114–19.
<<EPIC 3011>>

Shore, E R (1994). Outcomes of a primary prevention project for business and professional women. *Journal of Studies on Alcohol* **55**:657–9.
<<EPIC 3102>>

Sivyer, G, Gardiner, J, Hibbins, G and Saunders, R (1994). Smoking cessation study involving a transdermal nicotine patch: outcomes achieved in a workplace setting and in general practice. *Drug Investigation* **7**(5):244–53.
<<EPIC 3153>>

Sloan, R P (1990). Cessation and relapse in a year long workplace quit smoking contest. *Preventive Medicine* **19**(4):414–23.
<<EPIC 3042>>

Sorensen, G, Lando, H and Pechacek, T F (1993). Promoting smoking cessation at the workplace: results of a randomised controlled intervention study. *Journal of Occupational Medicine* **35**(2):121–6.
<<EPIC 3013>>

Sorensen, G, Beder, B, Prible, C R and Pinney, J (1995). Reducing smoking at the workplace: implementing a smoking ban and hypnotherapy. *Journal of Occupational and Environmental Medicine* **37**(4):453–60.
<<EPIC 3161>>

Takala, E, Viikari-Juntura, E and Tynkkynen, E (1994). Does group gymnastics at the workplace help in neck pain? *Scandinavian Journal of Rehabilitation Medicine* **26**:17–20.
<<EPIC 3099>>

Thompson, B, Emmons, K, Abrams, D, Ockene, J K and Feng, Z (1995a). ETS exposure in the workplace. *Journal of Occupational and Environmental Medicine* **37**(9):1086–92.
<<EPIC 3131>>

Thompson, B, Fries, E, Hopp, H, Bowen, D and Croyle, R (1995b). The feasibility of a proactive stepped care model for worksite smoking cessation. *Health Education Research* **10**(4):455–65.
<<EPIC 3157>>

Tregoning, D, Gent, N and Stephenson, D (1990). A comparison of the response of manual and non-manual workers to fitness testing. *Health Education Journal* **49**(1):30–1.
<<EPIC 3005>>

Walters, H, Bond, M and Pointer, S (1995). A stress management program for nursing home staff: an evaluation of combined education and relaxation strategies. *Journal of Occupational Health and Safety – Australia and New Zealand* **11**:243–8.
<<EPIC 3109>>

Weinberg, A D, Cooper, H P, Lane, M and Kripalani, S (1997). Screening behaviors and long-term compliance with mammography guidelines in a breast cancer screening program. *American Journal of Preventive Medicine* **13**(1):29–35.
<<EPIC 3110>>

Windsor, R A, Lowe, J B and Bartlett, E E (1988). The effectiveness of a worksite self-help smoking cessation program: a randomised trial. *Journal of Behavioral Medicine* **11**(4):407–21.
<<EPIC 3010>>

Wood, E, Olmstead, G and Craig, J (1989). An evaluation of lifestyle risk factors and absenteeism after two years in a worksite health promotion program. *American Journal of Health Promotion* **4**(2):128–33.
<<EPIC 3009>>

Woodruff, S I, Conway, T L and Bradway, L (1994). The US Navy Healthy Back Program: effect on back knowledge among recruits. *Military Medicine* **159**(7):475–84.
<<EPIC 3107>>

Zandee, G and Oermann, M (1996). Effectiveness of contingency contracting: component of a worksite weight loss program. *American Association of Occupational Health Nursing* **44**(4):183–8.
<<EPIC 3117>>

Zimmerman, R S, Safer, M A, Leventhal, H and Baumann, L J (1988). The effects of a worksite health promotion program on the wives of fire fighters. *Social Science and Medicine* **26**(5):537–43.
<<EPIC 3053>>

References

Action on Smoking and Health (ASH) (1993). *Her share of misfortune: women, smoking and low income.* London: ASH.

Alexy, B (1991). Factors associated with the participation or nonparticipation in a workplace wellness centre. *Research in Nursing and Health* **14**(1): 33–40

Anderson, D R and Staufacker, M J (1996). The impact of worksite-based health risk appraisal on health-related outcomes: a review of the literature. *American Journal of Health Promotion* **10**(6):499–508.

Baranowski, T, Henske, J, Simons-Morton, B *et al.* (1990). Dietary change for cardiovascular disease prevention among Black-American families. *Health Education Research* **5**(4):433–43.

Baun, W, Bernacki, E and Tsai, S (1986). A preliminary investigation: effect of a corporate fitness program on absenteeism and health care cost. *Journal of Occupational Medicine* **28**:18–22.

Biglan, A, Severson, H, Ary, D *et al.* (1987). Do smoking prevention programs really work? Attrition and the internal and external validity of an evaluation of an evaluation of a refusal skills training program. *Journal of Behavioral Medicine* **10**(2):159–71.

Blewett, V and Shaw, A (1995). Health promotion, handle with care: issues for health promotion in the workplace. *Journal of Occupational Health and Safety – Australia and New Zealand* **11**(5):461–5.

Boudreau, F, Godin, G, Pineau, R and Bradet, R (1995). Health risk appraisal in an occupational setting and its impact on exercise behavior. *Journal of Occupational and Environmental Medicine* **37**(9):1145–50.

Campbell, D T and Stanley, J C (1963). Experimental and quasi-experimental designs for research. Chicago: Rand McNally.

Carter, W B, Omenn, G S, Martin, M, Crump, C, Grunbaum, J A and Williams, O D (1995). Characteristics of health promotion programs in federal worksites: findings from the Federal Employee Worksite Project. *American Journal of Health Promotion* **10**(2):140–7.

Castillo-Salgado, C (1984). Assessing recent developments and opportunities in the promotion of health in the American workplace. *Social Science and Medicine* **19**(4):349–58.

Chalmers, I, Enkin, M and Keirse, M J (1989). *Effective care in pregnancy and childbirth.* Oxford: Oxford University Press.

Chalmers, I and Haynes, B (1994). Reporting, updating, and correcting systematic reviews of the effects of health care. *British Medical Journal* **309**:862–5.

Chalmers, T C, Celano, P, Sacks, H S and Smith, H (1983). Bias in treatment assignment in controlled clinical trials. *New England Journal of Medicine* **309**(22):1358–61.

Cirksena, M K and Flora, June A (1995). Audience segmentation in worksite health promotion: a procedure using social marketing concepts. *Health Education Research* **10**(2):211–24.

Clark, N and McLeroy, K (1995). Creating capacity through health education: what we know and what we don't know. *Health Education Quarterly* **22**(3):273–389.

Clarkson, J and Blower, E (1991). *Overview of innovative workplace action for health in the UK*. Dublin: European Foundation for the Improvement of Living and Working Conditions.

Cochrane Collaboration (1994). *Report*. Oxford: The Cochrane Centre.

Cochrane Library (1998). *The Cochrane Collaboration* (database on disk and CD-ROM). Oxford: Update Software.

Conrad, P (1987). Who comes to work-site wellness programs? A preliminary review. *Journal of Occupational Medicine* **29**(4):317–20.

Conrad, P (1988). Worksite health promotion: the social context. *Social Science and Medicine* **26**(5):485–9.

Cox, M, Shephard, R J and Corey, P (1981). Influence of an employee fitness programme upon fitness, productivity and absenteeism. *Ergonomics* **24**:795–806.

Coyle, S L, Boruch, R F and Turner, C F (1991). *Evaluating AIDS prevention programs*. Washington DC: National Academy Press.

Daley, A J and Parfitt, G (1996). Good health – is it worth it? Mood states, physical well-being, job satisfaction and absenteeism in members and non-members of a British corporate health and fitness club. *Journal of Occupational and Organizational Psychology* **69**(2):121–34.

Davis, K E, Jackson, K L, Kronenfeld, J J and Blair, S N (1987). Determinants of participation in worksite health promotion activities. *Health Education Quarterly* **14**(2):195–205.

Deacon, S (1996). Evaluate an occupational health programme. *Occupational Medicine* **46**(5):375–6.

Department of Health (1992). *The health of the nation: a strategy for health in England*. London: HMSO.

Department of Health and Human Services (DHHS) (1980). *Public Health Service: promoting health/preventing disease: objectives for the nation*. Washington DC: US Government Printing Office.

Dickersin, K and Lefebvre, C (1994). Identifying relevant studies for systematic reviews. *British Medical Journal* **309**:1286–91.

Donaldson, S I and Blanchard, A L (1995). The seven health practices, well-being and performance at work: evidence for the value of reaching small and underserved worksites. *Preventive Medicine* **24**:270–7.

Dugdill, L and Springett, J (1994). Evaluation of workplace health promotion: a review. *Health Education Journal* **53**:337–47.

Emmons, K, Linnan, L, Abrams, D and Lovell, H (1996). Women who work in manufacturing settings: factors, influencing their participation in worksite health promotion programs. *Women's Health Issues* **6**(2):74–81.

Erfurt, J C, Foote, A, Heirich, M A and Gregg, W (1990). Improving participation in worksite wellness programs: company health education classes, a menu approach, and follow-up counseling. *American Journal of Health Promotion* **4**:270–8.

 Faculty of Public Health Medicine. Committee on Health Promotion (1995). *Health promotion in the workplace*. Guidelines for Health Promotion No. 40. London: Royal Colleges of Physicians.

Fielding, J E (1990). Worksite health promotion programs in the United States: progress, lessons and challenges. *Health Promotion International* **5**(1):75–84.

Fielding, J E and Piserchia, P V (1989). Frequency of worksite health promotion activities. *American Journal of Public Health* **79**:16–20.

Fielding, J E, Mason, T, Knight, K, Klesges, R and Pelletier, K R (1995). A randomized trial of the IMPACT worksite cholesterol reduction program. *American Journal of Preventive Medicine* **11**(2):120–3.

Foshee, V, McLeroy, K R, Sumner, S K and Bibeau, D L (1986). Evaluation of worksite weight loss programs: a review of data and issues. *Journal of Nutrition Education* **18**(1):S38–S43.

France-Dawson, M, Holland, J, Fullerton, D, Kelly, P, Arnold, S and Oakley, A (1994). Review of effectiveness of workplace health promotion interventions. London: Social Science Research Unit.

Fullerton, D and Oakley, A (1995). *Young people and smoking.* London: Social Science Research Unit.

Gebhardt, D L and Crump, C E (1990). Employee fitness and wellness programs in the workplace. *American Psychology* **45**(2):262–72.

Glanz, K, Sorensen, G and Farmer, A (1996). The health impact of worksite nutrition and cholesterol intervention programs. *American Journal of Health Promotion* **10**(6):453–70.

Glasgow, R E, Hollis, J F, Ary, D V and Lando, H A (1990). Employee and organizational factors associated with participation in an incentive-based worksite smoking cessation program. *Journal of Behavioral Medicine* **13**:403–18.

Glasgow, R E, McCaul, K D and Fisher, K J (1993). Participation in worksite health promotion: a critique of the literature and recommendations for future practice. *Health Education Quarterly* **20**(3):391–408.

Goetzel, R Z, Kahr, T Y, Aldana, S G and Kenny, G M (1996). An evaluation of Duke University's Live for Life health promotion program and its impact on employee health. *American Journal of Health Promotion* **10**(5):340–1.

Green, L and Kreuter, M (1991). *Health promotion planning: an educational and environmental approach.* Mountain View, California: Mayfield Publishing Company.

Greene, G W and Strychar, I (1992). Participation in a worksite cholesterol education program in a university setting. *American Dietetic Association Journal* **92**(11):1376–81.

Hagard, S (1994). Health promotion at work [editorial]. *Promoting Education* **1**(1):3–5.

Hagard, S, Chambers, J and Killoran, A (1991). Health education in England: a five year strategy for the Health Education Authority. *Health Education Quarterly* **18**(1):49–63.

Hawe, P, Degeling, D and Hall, J (1995). *Evaluating health promotion: a health worker's guide.* Sydney: MacLennan & Petty.

Health Education Authority (1993). *Health promotion in the workplace – a summary.* London: HEA.

Heaney, C A and Inglish, P (1995). Are employees who are at risk for cardiovascular disease joining worksite fitness centers? *Journal of Occupational and Environmental Medicine* **37**(6):718–24.

Heaney, C A and Goldenhar, L M (1996). Worksite health programs: working together to advance employee health (introduction). *Health Education Quarterly* **23**(2):133–6.

Hennrikus, D J and Jeffery, R W (1996). Worksite intervention for weight control: a review of the literature. *American Journal of Health Promotion* **10**(6):471–98.

Hollander, R B and Lengermann, J J (1988). Corporate characteristics and worksite health promotion programs: survey findings from Fortune 500 companies. *Social Science and Medicine* **26**(5):491–501.

Homans, H and Aggleton, P (1989). Health education, HIV infection and AIDS. In: Aggleton, P and Homans, H (eds). *Social aspects of AIDS.* Lewes: Falmer Press, pp. 154–76.

Ingledew, D (1986). All work and no play. *Health Service Journal* **6**:1162–3.

Israel, B, Cummings, K, Dignan, M, Heaney, C, Perales, D, Simons-Morton B and Zimmerman, M (1995). Evaluation of health education programs: current assessment and future directions. *Health Education Quarterly* **22**(3):364–89.

Jacobsen, B, Smith, A and Whitehead, M (1991). *The nation's health: a strategy for the 1990s.* London: King's Fund.

Jeffery, R W, Kelder, S H, Forster, J L, French, S A, Lando, H A and Baxter, J E (1994). Restrictive smoking policies in the workplace: effects on smoking prevalence and cigarette consumption. *Preventive Medicine* **23**:78–82.

Karasek, R and Theorell, T (1990). *Healthy work: stress, productivity, and the reconstruction of working life.* London: Harper Collins.

Knight, K K, Goetzel, R Z, Fielding, J E, Eisen, M, Jackson, G W, Kahr, T Y, Kenny, G M, Wade, S W and Duann, S (1994). An evaluation of Duke University's Live For Life health promotion program on changes in worker absenteeism. *Journal of Occupational and Environmental Medicine* **36**(5):533–6.

Knipschild, P (1994). Systematic reviews: some examples. *British Medical Journal* **309**:719–21.

Kogan, H (1996). Oh: a jack of all trades? *Occupational Health* **48**(1):10.

Labour Research Department (1989). *Workplace health – a trade unionist's guide.* London: LRO Publications.

Lerman, Y and Shemer, J (1996). Epidemiologic characteristics of participants and nonparticipants in health-promotion programs. *Journal of Occupational and Environmental Medicine* **38**(5):535–8.

Loevinsohn, B P (1990). Health education interventions in developing countries: a methodological review of published articles. *International Journal of Epidemiology* **4**:788–94.

Lusk, S L, Kerr, M J and Ronis, D L (1995). Health-promoting lifestyles of blue-collar, skilled trade, and white-collar workers. *Nursing Research* **44**(1):20–4.

MacDonald, G, Sheldon, B and Gillespie, J (1992). Contemporary studies of the effectiveness of social work. *British Journal of Social Work* **22**(6):615–43.

Macdonald, S and Wells, S (1995). Lifestyle problems and health programs in Ontario worksectors. *Employee Assistance Quarterly* **11**(2):37–50.

Mittlemark, M B, Luepker, R V, Jacobs, D R *et al.* (1989). A community-wide prevention of cardiovascular disease: education strategies of the Minnesota Heart Health Program. *Preventive Medicine* **15**:1–17.

Mulrow, C D (1994). Rationale for systematic reviews. *British Medical Journal* **309**:597–9.

Nutbeam, D and Catford, J (1987). The Welsh Heart programme evaluation strategy: progress, plans and possibilities. *Health Promotion* **2**(1):5–18.

Oakley, A (1998). Experimentation in social science: the case of health promotion. *Social Sciences in Health* (in press) **4**(2):73–89.

Oakley, A and Fullerton, D (1994). *Risk, knowledge and behaviour: HIV/AIDS education programmes and young people.* London: Social Science Research Unit.

Oakley, A and Fullerton, D (1996). The lamp-post of research: support or illumination? In: Oakley, A and Roberts, H (eds). *Evaluating social interventions.* London: Barnardos.

Oakley, A, Fullerton, D, Holland, J, Arnold, S, France-Dawson, M, Kelly, P, McGrellis, S and Robertson, P (1994a). *Reviews of effectiveness: sexual health interventions for young people.* London: Social Science Research Unit.

Oakley, A, Fullerton, D, Holland, J, Arnold, S, Hickey, D, Kelley, P, McGrellis, S and Robertson, P (1994b). *Towards effective interventions: a critical evaluation of HIV prevention and sexual health education interventions*. London: Social Science Research Unit.

Oakley, A, Fullerton, D and Holland, J (1995). Behavioral interventions for HIV AIDS-prevention. *AIDS*:**9**(5): 479–86.

Oakley, A, Fullerton, D, Holland, J, Arnold, S, France-Dawson, M, Kelly, P and McGrellis, S (1995a). Sexual health education interventions for young people: a methodological review. *British Medical Journal* **310**:158–62.

Oakley, A, France-Dawson, M, Fullerton, D, Holland, J and Arnold, S (in collaboration with the South East Institute of Public Health) (1995b). *Review of effectiveness of health promotion interventions to prevent accidents in older people*. London: Social Science Research Unit.

Oakley, A, Oliver, S, Peersman, G and Mauthner, M (1996). *Review of effectiveness of health promotion interventions for men who have sex with men*. London: EPI-Centre, Social Science Research Unit.

O'Donnell, M P (1987). Design of workplace health promotion programs. *American Journal of Health Promotion* **3**:1–47.

Office of Population Censuses and Surveys (OPCS) (1992). *General Household Survey 1990*. An interdepartmental survey carried out by OPCS between April 1990 and March 1991. London: HMSO.

Parker, G (1996). General practitioners and occupational health services. *British Journal of General Practice* **46**(406):303–5.

Peersman, G, Oakley, A, Oliver, S and Thomas, J (1996). *Review of effectiveness of sexual health promotion interventions for young people*. London: EPI-Centre, Social Science Research Unit.

Pelletier, K R (1993). A review and analysis of the health and cost-effective outcome studies of comprehensive health promotion and disease prevention programs at the worksite: 1991–1993 update. *American Journal of Health Promotion* **8**(1):50–62.

Pelletier, K R (1991). A review and analysis of the health and cost effective outome studies of comprehensive health promotion and disease prevention programs. *American Journal of Health Promotion* **5**(4):311–13.

Pencak, M (1991). Workplace health promotion programs. *Nursing Clinic of North America* **26**(1):233–40.

Potter, J D, Graves, K L, Finnegan, J R *et al.* (1990). The cancer and diet intervention project: a community-based intervention to reduce nutrition-related risk of cancer. *Health Education Research* **5**(4):489–503.

Reason, J (1989). *The LAYH Workplace Initiative – a progress report*. London: Health Education Authority.

Roman, P M and Blum, T C (1996). Alcohol: a review of the impact of worksite interventions on health and behavioral outcomes. *American Journal of Health Promotion* **11**(2):136–49.

Sadler, S and Thomas, M (1994). Workplace health: surveying employers' attitudes. *Occupational Health* **46**(8):272–4.

Sanders, D and Crowe, S (1996). Overview of health promotion in the workplace. In: Scriven, A and Orme, J (eds). *Health promotion: professional perspectives*. London: Macmillan, pp. 199–209.

Sapolsky, H M, Altman, D, Greene, R and Moore, J B (1981). Corporate attitudes towards health care costs. *Milbank Memorial Fund Quarterly/Health and Society* **59**:561–85.

Schnaps, E, De Bartolo, R, Moskowitz, J, Pally, C S and Churgin, S (1981). A review of 127 drug prevention program evaluations. *Journal of Drug Issues* **11**:17–43.

Schwartz, D, Flamant, R and Lellouch, J (1980). *Clinical trials*. London: Academic Press.

Sepulveda, M, Goetz, A and Grana, J (1994). Measuring second-order selection bias in a work site health program. *Journal of Occupational Medicine* **36**(3):326–33.

Shephard, R J (1996). Worksite fitness and exercise programs: a review of methodology and health impact. *American Journal of Health Promotion* **10**(6):436–52.

Silverman, W A (1985). *Human experimentation: a guided step into the unknown*. Oxford: Oxford Medical Publications.

Sorensen, G, Pechacek, T and Pallonen, U (1986). Occupational and worksite norms and attitudes about smoking cessation. *American Journal of Public Health* **76**:544–9.

Sorensen, G, Stoddard, A, Ockene, J K, Hunt, M K and Youngstrom, R (1996). Worker participation in an integrated health promotion/health protection program: results from the WellWorks Project. *Health Education Quarterly* **23**(2):191–203.

Speller, V, Learmonth, A and Harrison, D (1997). The search for evidence of effective health promotion. *British Medical Journal* **315**:361–3.

Spilman, M A (1988). Gender differences in worksite health promotion activities. *Social Science and Medicine* **26**(5):525–35.

Springett, J and Dugdill, L (1995). Workplace health promotion programmes: towards a framework for evaluation. *Health Education Journal* **54**:88–98.

Stachnik, T and Stoffelmayr, B (1983). Worksite smoking cessation programs: a potential for national impact. *American Journal of Public Health* **73**(12):1395–6.

Stokols, D, Pelletier, K and Fielding, J (1995). Integration of medical care and worksite health promotion. *Journal of the American Medical Association* **273**(14):1136–42.

Stunkard, A J, Cohen, R Y and Felix, M R J (1989). Weight loss competitions at the worksite: how they work and how well. *Preventive Medicine* **18**:460–74.

Townsend, P and Davidson, N (eds) (1982). *Inequalities in health – the Black Report*. London: Penguin Books.

Townsend, P, Davidson, N and Whitehead, M (eds) (1988). *Inequalities in health: 'The Black Report' and 'The Health Divide'*. London: Penguin Books.

Tregoning, D, Gent, N and Stephenson, D (1990). A comparison of the response of manual and non-manual workers to fitness testing. *Health Education Journal* **49**(1):30–1.

Walsh, D C, Jennings, S E, Mangione, T and Merrigan, D M (1991). Health promotion versus health protection? Employees' perceptions and concerns. *Journal of Public Health Policy* **12**(2):148–64.

Weinstein, M S (1983). *Health promotion and lifestyle change in the worksite*. Copenhagen: WHO European Regional Office.

Whitehead, M (1987). *The health divide: inequalities in health in the 1980s*. London: Health Education Council.

Wilbur, C S (1983). Live for Life: the Johnson & Johnson program. *Preventive Medicine* **12**:672–81.

Wilson, M G, Holman, P B and Hammock, A (1996). A comprehensive review of the effects of worksite health promotion on health-related outcomes. *American Journal of Health Promotion* **10**(6):429–35.

Wilson, M G, Jorgensen, C and Cole, G (1996). The health effects of worksite HIV/AIDS interventions: a review of the research literature. *American Journal of Health Promotion* **11**(2):150–7.

Wong, M L, Alsagoff, F and Koh, D (1992). Health promotion – a further field to conquer. *Singapore Medical Journal* **33**(4):341–6.

Zaslow, M J and Takanishi, R (1993). Priorities for research on adolescent development. *American Psychology* **48**:185–92.

Zavela, K J, Davis, L G, Cottrell, R R and Smith, W E (1988). Do only the healthy intend to participate in worksite health promotion? *Health Education Quarterly* **15**:259–67.

Maintaining and raising the standards of systematic reviews

This review collates evidence about effectiveness intended to help people make better decisions about health promotion. It is obviously important that every effort (within the resources available) is made to ensure that the sources of information and methods used to collate evidence of effectiveness maximise the likely validity of the review's conclusions.

Anyone wishing to suggest how methods for systematically reviewing health promotion literature may be improved, or able to comment on judgements made during this review is invited to contact the EPI-Centre.

EPI-Centre
Social Science Research Unit
London University Institute of Education
18 Woburn Square
London WC1H 0NS

Tel: +44 171 612 6816
Fax:+44 171 612 6400
E-mail:health@ioe.ac.uk